Praise for *DIY Autoflowering Cannabis*

For the first time, short-blooming cannabis varieties are available
in seed form that put easy cannabis growing within reach of gardeners
anywhere in the United States. Jeff Lowenfels' *DIY Autoflowering
Cannabis* provides everything you need to source seeds,
grow, and harvest your first cannabis plants!

SHANGO LOS Shaping Fire Podcast

DIY Autoflowering Cannabis is an approachable and necessary
guide for dedicated beginners and gardening ninjas alike. Lowenfels'
book is the ultimate course load: history, biology, chemistry, Latin *and*
home use (yes, there are recipes!). Readers are actually encouraged to
skip class to experience things first hand. I learned an incredible
amount about autoflowering cannabis—better yet, I was inspired.

JULES TORTI editor-in-chief, *Harrowsmith* magazine, and author,
Free to a Good Home: With Room for Improvement

DIY Autoflowering Cannabis is *the* book to read for anyone who
wants to be at the forefront of cannabis cultivation. Jeff Lowenfels weaves
together the science and hands-on cultivation of this new breed of
cannabis into an informative, enjoyable, and often humorous, good read.

LEE REICH PhD, scientist, farmdener (more than a gardener,
less than a farmer), and author, *The Ever Curious Gardener*

At last, something easier and faster, *and* gentler than habanero peppers to satisfy our lust for home-grown satisfaction. Always loved Jeff's plain-spoken enthusiasms, but this easy, beautiful book is a fantastic inspiration for enjoying this alluring breakthrough plant!

FELDER RUSHING NPR host and founder, Slow Gardening

Jeff Lowenfels is the best go-to author for cannabis information that I know. At a time when the internet is filled with myths, rumors, or downright inaccurate information about this plant, Jeff provides accurate, useful, and accessible advice that all cannabis growers can use.

C.L. FORNARI author and co-host, Plantrama Podcast

It's an honor to have such a legendary author write an entire book on a plant so near and dear to our hearts! We commend you Jeff for bringing the attention of others to this amazing plant that we love so much! The use of plant history, growing information, and garden humor makes this book an enjoyable gateway to the autoflowering cannabis plant that can be enjoyed by anyone!

MEPHISTO GENETICS

DIY

AUTOFLOWERING

CANNABIS

AN EASY WAY TO GROW YOUR OWN

JEFF LOWENFELS

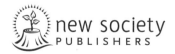

new society
PUBLISHERS

Inquiries regarding requests to reprint all or part of DIY *Autoflowering Cannabis* should be addressed to New Society Publishers at the address below. To order directly from the publishers, please call toll-free (North America) 1-800-567-6772, or order online at www.newsociety.com

Any other inquiries can be directed by mail to:
New Society Publishers
P.O. Box 189, Gabriola Island, BC VOR 1X0, Canada
(250) 247-9737

LIBRARY AND ARCHIVES CANADA CATALOGUING IN PUBLICATION

Title: DIY auto-flowering cannabis : an easy way to grow your own! / by Jeff Lowenfels.
Other titles: Do it yourself auto-flowering cannabis
Names: Lowenfels, Jeff, author.
Description: Includes index.

Identifiers: Canadiana (print) 20190145153 | Canadiana (ebook) 20190145161 |
    ISBN 9780865719163 (softcover) | ISBN 9781550927085 (PDF) |
    ISBN 9781771423045 (EPUB)

Subjects: LCSH: Cannabis—Propagation—Handbooks, manuals, etc. | LCSH: Marijuana—Handbooks, manuals, etc. | LCSH: Gardening—Handbooks, manuals, etc. | LCGFT: Handbooks and manuals.

Classification: LCC SB295.C35 L69 2019 | DDC 633.7/9—dc23

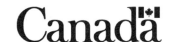

Funded by the Government of Canada
Financé par le gouvernement du Canada

New Society Publishers' mission is to publish books that contribute in fundamental ways to building an ecologically sustainable and just society, and to do so with the least possible impact on the environment, in a manner that models this vision.

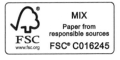

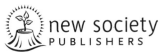

FSC MIX Paper from responsible sources FSC® C016245

Certified B Corporation

new society PUBLISHERS

▶ Seedling GBD/DAZ MEPHISTO GENETICS

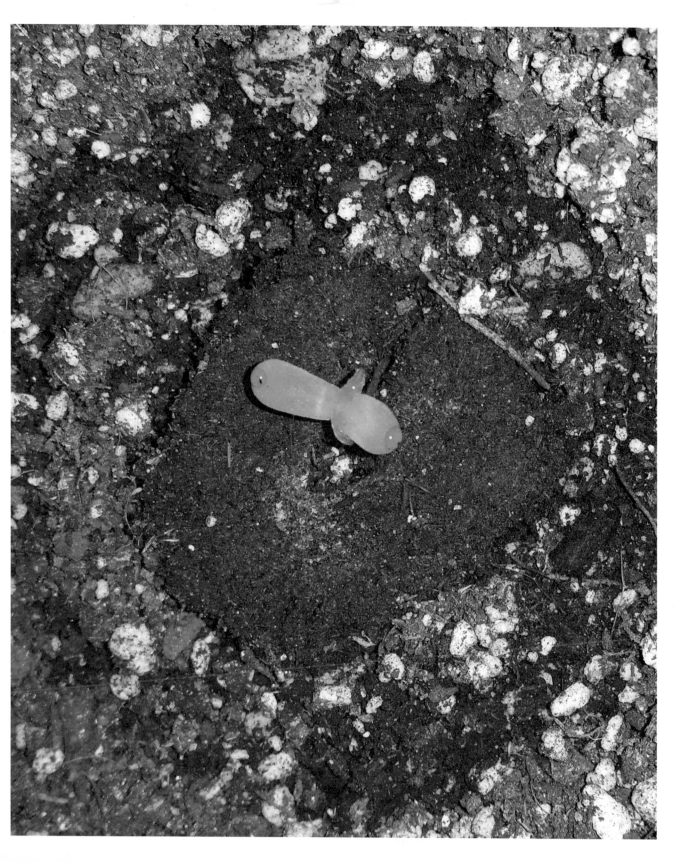

CONTENTS

ACKNOWLEDGMENTS

S O MANY THANKS to Judith Hoersting for letting me go into the writer's rabbit hole and putting up with me. Kudos to Harold Frazier at New Breed Seed, Fred Gunnerson at SoFreshFarms, Gdb/Daz at Mephisto Genetics, Sebring Frehner, and Full Duplex for their help and fantastic photos.

This book is dedicated to Tom Alexander,
unsung hero for all he has done for
the cannabis movement, and for kindling
my interest in Autoflowering Cannabis,
the next tomato!

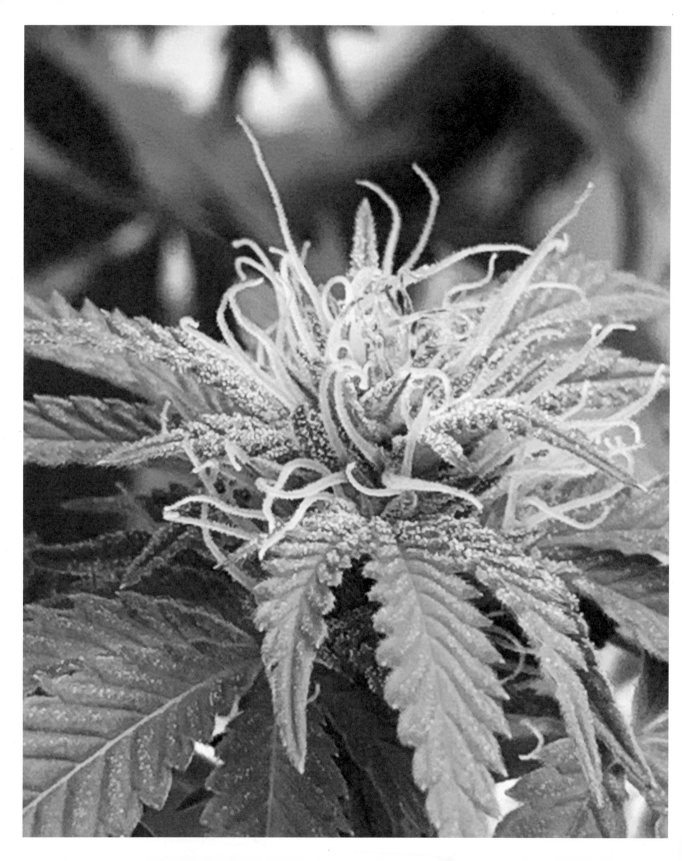

PREFACE

DIY AUTOFLOWERING CANNABIS, *An Easy Way to Grow Your Own*, introduces a brand new plant to gardeners, one that is easy to grow, beautiful, and useful too: Autoflowering *Cannabis*. Why me and why Autoflowering *Cannabis*? I have been writing a newspaper garden column every single week (without fail) for nearly 45 years. If there is one thing I have learned from writing all those columns, it is that gardeners, even the most casual, are always looking for something new and different to grow.

This is why breeding new plants for the home gardener is a huge industry. Every spring, new varieties of roses, pansies, petunias, hydrangeas, and more appear in box stores, greenhouses, and nurseries. For most gardeners, the new plant introductions are the best part of the catalogs that come out each year. However, it isn't often that a *whole new category* of plants becomes available to the home gardener.

Now that *Cannabis* prohibition is ending, you would think there would be lots of interest in growing *Cannabis* in home gardens, and on porches and decks. Unfortunately, there are a number of really big obstacles that prevent regular *Cannabis* from becoming a popular home garden plant.

First, the biggest barrier is that regular *Cannabis* plants are dependent on daylength to bloom. Actually, it is night length, but either way, this is known as photoperiodism. Nights must be more

▶ Flower HAROLD FRAZIER, NEW BREED SEED

than 12 hours before flowering will start, and it is the flowers that are harvested.

This is not a problem in and of itself, but shortening days are accompanied by cooler weather in most places around the world. In many, frosts kill the plants before they are ready to harvest.

Not so with Autoflowering *Cannabis*! Autoflowers (for short, also called Day-Neutral *Cannabis* and, sometimes, Automatic *Cannabis*) do not flower based on a photoperiod. They can flower anytime, indoors or outdoors, regardless of how long (or short) nights happen to be.

This kind of *Cannabis* evolved in Northern climes where the growing season is extremely short. To survive, plants must grow very fast and produce viable seeds before they are killed by the chill. Over time, some evolved so that genetics trigger timely flowering, not a change in photoperiod.

As a result, home gardeners who grow Autoflowering *Cannabis* don't have to worry about-immature plants being taken down prematurely. I garden in short season Alaska, so I know this firsthand.

Moreover, since Autoflowering *Cannabis* is not triggered into flowering by light or darkness, gardeners don't have to worry, as do regular *Cannabis* growers, about street lights or someone accidently interrupting a dark period by turning on lights.

The second major problem with regular photoperiod *Cannabis* is that these are normally really big plants, some reaching 3 meters (10 feet) or more high (sorry) and just as wide. These are much larger than the casual gardener can handle. They certainly don't fit on an apartment or condo deck.

Once again, Autoflowering *Cannabis* has it covered. These plants are much, much smaller than their cousins. Some are Lilliputian and only get 30 to 45 cm (12 to 18 inches) tall! Others can grow to about 90 cm (3 feet), still a size perfectly suited for growing in containers, outdoors on a deck, or indoors under lights.

Now, photoperiod and smaller plants would be quite enough to convince many to grow Autoflowering *Cannabis*, but there is one more convincing factor. Larger regular varieties of *Cannabis* can take several months and more to flower. Often seeds started in April don't produce until December or January (or even later). Not only would this try the patience of a home gardener, but as earlier noted, in most cases cold weather would take them down. Growing *Cannabis* is limited to those that have a long enough growing season or an indoor growing area.

Ah, but Autoflowers start flowering after only 2 to 3 weeks and can often be harvested after as little as 7 to 8 weeks. There is no problem getting at least one outdoor crop each summer, and an indoor gardener can grow them anytime of the year.

To add to all of this, Autoflowering *Cannabis* plants have now been bred to produce the same level of chemicals for which commercially grown regular *Cannabis* is famous. This makes it possible for the home gardener to grow useable *Cannabis* instead of buying it.

These plants, minus the chemicals, are surprising similar to tomatoes. In fact, I often compare the two plants, as you will see! The point is, if you can grow tomatoes, you can quickly learn to grow Autoflowering *Cannabis*. (Here is where I should make a lame joke about Autoflowering *Cannabis* as the new stewed tomatoes.)

There are lots of other attributes to Autoflowers that will entice the hobby gardener. However, at the top of the list, Autoflowering *Cannabis* plants are very easy to grow once you become familiar with them. In addition, they are attractive plants that usually have a delightful smell. And, you can breed your own, just as you might develop your own heirloom tomatoes.

So, for gardeners who are looking for something new and different to grow, here it is! Autoflowering *Cannabis* is a brand-new category of plants that are easy for any gardener to grow, from casual to expert.

There are a myriad of *Cannabis* books covering the photoperiod type. Many of these are coffee-table books with fantastic pictures I call bud porn. Others are written for would-be commercial growers. Often they are kept under lock and key at book stores, for some unjustified reason.

This book, however, is a very simple guide to get gardeners started and to lead them into the hobby of growing Autoflowering *Cannabis* at home. The text is predicated on the notion that you are an *organic gardener*.

By gardener, I mean that you know how to water a plant, that it needs proper light, and what to monitor to know when things are not going right. If you have never grown plants, fine, but you might need some very basic growing instructions that I don't provide here.

By organic, I mean you use what nature has given us via soil, not synthetic chemicals. After all, if you are going to grow Autoflowering *Cannabis*, you are probably going to ingest it. For this reason alone, you need to make sure yours is safe to consume. Growing organically is the best way to be sure.

If you are not already an organic gardener, I urgently point you toward a trilogy of books I have written on the subject. Dangerous chemicals have no place in a hobby situation. *Teaming with Microbes: The Organic Gardener's Guide to the Soil Food Web* (Timber Press, 2006) will introduce you to the science of organics and the soil food web. It is crucial to your understanding of how an organic system should work.

Teaming with Fungi: The Organic Grower's Guide to Mycorrhizae (Timber Press, 2017) is about mycorrhizal fungi, which are all-important for feeding plants. And, speaking of feeding plants, *Teaming with Nutrients: The Organic Gardener's Guide to Optimizing Plant Nutrition* (Timber Press, 2013) is all about what plants need to eat, from an organic perspective, and how they use the nutrients.

All three of my books will help you be a better organic gardener. They are used by many commercial *Cannabis* growers all around the globe. They will also help you grow better Autoflowering *Cannabis*.

A word or two about pictures: I wanted to include a million pictures but could not due to page limitations. So I opted to limit bud porn here and left out pictures of obvious supplies, or accents to the history mentioned and the like, as you can easily find these elsewhere. You can and should resort to the Internet to see what is out there.

Finally, and by all means most important, I want you to realize that growing Autoflowering *Cannabis* plants is just like gardening with any other plant. Nothing more.

We are discussing gardening as a hobby and not as an occupation. As such, it is supposed to be fun and enjoyable, not stressful work. I can assure you that once you start gardening with Autoflowering *Cannabis*, you will soon see what makes them so fascinating to me and why I have come to believe that they will be the home gardener's next tomato.

1

SOMETHING TOTALLY NEW FOR THE HOME GARDENER

CONGRATULATIONS! YOU ARE embarking on growing something totally new to home gardeners, Autoflowering *Cannabis*. These are special plants developed as a way to improve upon the attributes of its parents, *Cannabis sativa*, *indica*, and *ruderalis*. The history of this development will give you an appreciation of what these plants are, what they can do, and what you should expect. This all adds up to why you should grow them.

Cannabis originated in Central and South Asia where it has grown at least since the Neolithic period, some 10,000 or so years, BC. By 500 BC, Russian, Japanese, and Chinese craftsmen were growing and using *Cannabis* plants to produce cloth as well as rope. These plants were probably not psychoactive, though they were most probably used as medicine.

GROWING *CANNABIS* IS NOT NEW

Somewhere along the way, the plant's psychoactive properties were discovered (and probably increased by breeding methods), though the importance of this was limited to religious ceremonies (and, surely, the occasional farmer who grew a variety that allowed family and close friends to indulge). It was *Cannabis's* ability to be made into rope, cloth, and paper that mattered.

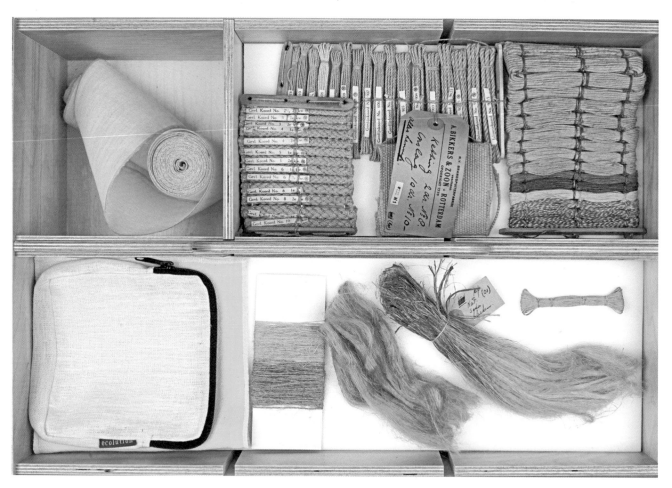

▲ Hemp has many uses as a result of its fibrous nature and can be made into fiber, paper, yarn, textile, and rope. JOEP VOGELS, TEXTIELMUSEUM TILBURG - WIKICOMMONS.

Cannabis was so important that, in 1619, the North American colony of Virginia passed a law requiring all farmers to grow *Cannabis sativa* (L.), the variety of *Cannabis* that is known as hemp. A similar tax law was instituted in the colonies of Massachusetts and then Connecticut. In some colonies, hemp was even accepted as currency. The end result is that the US Constitution was written on hemp paper.

For about 150 years after the US Revolution, hemp was the United States' largest single cash crop. In the early 1800s, in order to stimulate production, the Canadian government started to give out hemp seed to farmers. These efforts were successful in starting a Canadian hemp industry.

Today there are all manner of stories, most of them true, about the use of *Cannabis* by famous Americans and Canadians. The most famous of these is that as a tax-paying Virginian, George Washington, even while President of the United States, grew *Cannabis*. (Or, rather, the slaves he owned did.)

NORTH AMERICA STOPPED GROWING *CANNABIS*

In the early to mid-1900s, *Cannabis* use was stigmatized. In 1923, without a shard of scientific evidence, it was made illegal in Canada, a move precipitated by a lone Federal Narcotics Director who had just returned from a League of Nations session where the issue had been debated.

The change in Canadian law happened almost by accident and very late at night. There is scant record of what happened or why, unlike in the United States. There, a desperate Harry Jacob Anslinger, the head of the US bureau that oversaw alcohol prohibition, created and then conducted a relentless, racially biased campaign against *Cannabis*.

You can look up the rest of the story. Anslinger used racism and fake news (he was one of the best at it) to make the case for prohibition of *Cannabis*. There was absolutely no science involved.

In the 1960s, US President Richard Nixon's administration played a role in *Cannabis* prohibition, again with no science and only politics as support. Even the wife of President Ronald Regan, a few years later, added to the nonsensical treatment of *Cannabis*.

There was even pressure put on border crossings between the United States and Canada. All of a sudden, a lot of people in both countries and the rest of the world were being arrested for possessing a plant, even though there was no scientific reason for such actions.

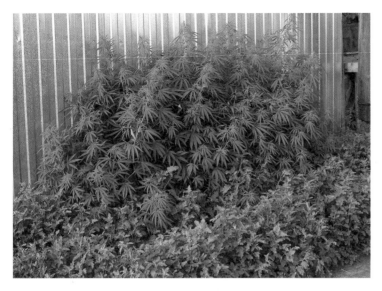

▲ Maturing wild *Cannabis* plants (*Cannabis sativa* var. *ruderalis* Janisch; syn. *Cannabis ruderalis* Janisch) and *Atriplex tatarica* on a private driveway in Saratov City, Russia. LE.LOUP.GRIS, WIKICOMMONS.

CANNABIS MAKES A COMEBACK

This is a book on how to grow a plant, not a book about politics. It is enough to note that there has been a sea change in attitudes about *Cannabis* in North America and the rest of the world. Hence the ability to publish these words so openly.

It is now legal to grow *Cannabis* in Canada and in many of the United States. More and more states and countries throughout the world are decriminalizing possession of *Cannabis*. As a result of all of this liberalization, a huge commercial *Cannabis* industry is developing.

For the most part (setting aside exact genetic science for a simpler explanation), plants used by commercial *Cannabis* growers are of the two main types, *Cannabis sativa* and *Cannabis indica*. The former evolved to grow in equatorial areas. These are slow growers that get very tall. The latter originated in the Indian subcontinent. These are shorter and flower just a bit earlier.

The first time I saw an Autoflowering *Cannabis* plant was in the late 1970s. It was my first Lowryder, the successful result of early crosses between regular *Cannabis* and *Cannabis ruderalis*. It was a dream come true for hobby growers.

The diminutive size of this new form of *Cannabis* was of great interest. It could be grown safely hidden in the tiniest and least likely of places to be discovered. And the speed with which the plant developed was astounding! Seven weeks from seed to harvest was simply a dream. The odds of some authority like your parents stumbling onto your crop were greatly reduced.

Add to all of this, completing the dream, no photoperiod required! This was freedom from seasonality. It almost didn't matter that the THC content of this plant was not as high as experienced with the *sativas* and *indicas* of the day.

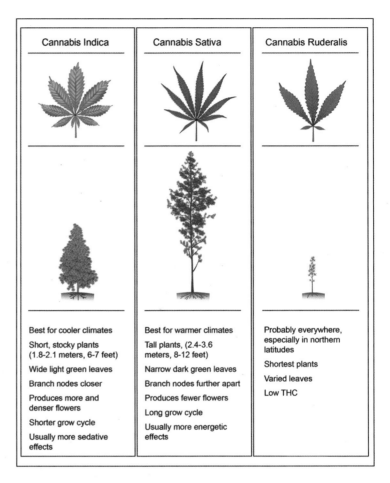

Cannabis Indica	Cannabis Sativa	Cannabis Ruderalis
Best for cooler climates	Best for warmer climates	Probably everywhere, especially in northern latitudes
Short, stocky plants (1.8-2.1 meters, 6-7 feet)	Tall plants, (2.4-3.6 meters, 8-12 feet)	Shortest plants
Wide light green leaves	Narrow dark green leaves	Varied leaves
Branch nodes closer	Branch nodes further apart	Low THC
Produces more and denser flowers	Produces fewer flowers	
Shorter grow cycle	Long grow cycle	
Usually more sedative effects	Usually more energetic effects	

Sativa versus Indica versus Ruderalis Cannabis

▲ Illustration of the three main types of *Cannabis*. WINNIE CASACOP.

Fortunately, both of these photoperiod *Cannabis* plants can cross with a third type, *Cannabis ruderalis*. The word *ruderalis* is an adjectival form of the Latin word for rubble. These plants are found in previously disturbed poor soil. The original plants are the evolved offspring of *Cannabis sativa* that developed in high-altitude regions of Russia where the growing season is very short.

Cannabis ruderalis plants are day-neutral, naturally autoflowering. They are low in psychoactive chemicals but can cross with *Cannabis sativa* and *Cannabis indica*. Resultant seed can have *Cannabis ruderalis's* ability to flower based solely on genetic maturity and not daylength. They can also have the higher potency mix of chemicals for which the bigger plants are grown.

DEVELOPMENT OF AUTOFLOWERING *CANNABIS*

Add together the diminutive size of *ruderalis* plants plus their fast-growing characteristics, and all of a sudden you have bred a new plant variety that can be easily grown at home! It grows fast in any photoperiod, doesn't need great soil, and is small in size when it comes to *Cannabis*.

Breeding efforts continued to bear fruit (actually, seeds), resulting in smaller plants, 60 cm (2 feet) or less, which could be grown from seed to harvest in only 7 to 9 weeks. They are perfect for growing at home, on a deck, or indoors.

A second type of plant was developed, known as, loosely, Super Autoflowering *Cannabis*. These are slightly larger plants that produce a higher (oops, better use larger) yield but can take 100 days to grow, which is still very short for *Cannabis*.

While their relatively larger size may discourage a few indoor home gardeners who don't have as much room in which to grow them, Super Autoflowers are fine for outdoor garden or deck gardeners. In fact, more and more commercial growers are using them because at least they don't have to worry about daylength and frosts.

There are advantages to growing either type of Autoflowering *Cannabis*. If you lack space entirely, consider the smaller kind. If you want more yield, go with the Supers.

GROWING AUTOFLOWERING *CANNABIS*
REALLY IS A LOT LIKE GROWING TOMATOES

From my experience, growing Autoflowering *Cannabis* is very much like growing tomatoes. I don't make this comparison lightly. As with

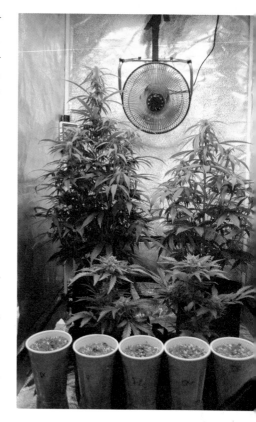

▲ Unlike their cousins, Autoflowering *Cannabis*, foreground, are small plants. However, breeding efforts have resulted in larger Super Autoflowering *Cannabis* plants like the taller ones here. SEBRING FREHNER.

tomatoes, Autoflowering *Cannabis* plants are really easy to germinate and grow. The plant does almost all of the work. The harvest is useable and enjoyable and one which you will probably never become tired of, unlike with zucchini or kale.

You can grow Autoflowers from germination to harvest in as little as 7 to 8 weeks. That is about the time you can get first early tomatoes. Autoflowering *Cannabis* plants have tomatoes beat, however, as they start to flower after only 2 or 3 weeks. This makes them easy, easy, easy to grow, while tomatoes are just easy, easy.

The analogy to tomatoes breaks down when it comes to the goal of growing *Cannabis*. It is the production of flowers that contain medicinal and recreational qualities for which *Cannabis* is known. With tomatoes, it is the fruit formed *after* the flowers.

However, to get back on track with comparing both plants, a gardener can easily end up growing the proverbial 40-dollar tomato. A lot of money can be wasted growing a plant that produces poorly. There is an Autoflowering *Cannabis* equivalent, but that is only if you don't know what you are doing, which is what this book is for.

And, just as the tomato can be grown for its contribution to nutritional health (in part because of the interesting chemistry of the lycopene it contains), there are medicinal values to Autoflowering *Cannabis* plants as a result of equally interesting chemistry. As more research is completed as a result of legalization, more health benefits are being discovered or confirmed.

Finally, home gardeners can produce homegrown Autoflowering seeds, just as we do with tomatoes (though there is a difference explained later). You can develop your own strains of Autoflowering *Cannabis* just as you can develop your own heritage or heirloom tomatoes. This makes growing Autoflowering *Cannabis* a really multifaceted horticultural hobby.

EASY TO GROW ONCE YOU KNOW THE ROPES

Once again (and it won't be the last reminder), growing Autoflowering *Cannabis*, like growing tomatoes, is easy. With both, you stick a seed into damp soil, and you most probably get a plant, even if you do nothing else but water. You may not get *good* tomatoes or *many Cannabis* flowers, but you will have some harvest unless you kill the plant.

Ah, but who wants just a plant? If you are a gardener, you want the best plant you can grow. In short, as my Dad taught me (though he did not approve of *Cannabis*, that is for sure!), there is vast difference between growing an easy plant and growing an easy plant properly. This is where *DIY AutoFlowering Cannabis: An Easy Way to Grow Your Own* comes in.

If you want lots of flavorful tomatoes, you need to prune and feed properly, stake correctly, and make sure there is effective pollination. Still, there is not a lot of work involved. The same goes with successfully growing Autoflowering *Cannabis* plants. However, they grow so fast that it isn't enough to just know what the plants need; you need to know when they need it as well.

They are new to you now, but Autoflowering *Cannabis* plants are simply plants, and like any plant, getting the cultural information you need and growing it is all it takes. Once you finish the next chapters, you will be on your way.

LEGALITY

Cannabis legalization doesn't mean growing *Cannabis,* even the autoflowering kind, is free of restrictions. Your jurisdiction may limit the number of plants you can grow at one time. Or you may be limited to the amount of *Cannabis* in general that you are allowed to possess at any given time.

The bottom line, if you are going to grow Autoflowering *Cannabis,* make sure you know what the rules are in your jurisdiction. Obey them.

ROAD MAP

This book will first cover a bit of the special chemistry and botany associated with all *Cannabis* plants. This will be simple and broad-brushed and is included because I need to make sure we are using the same terms and you know what (and where) to look as the plant develops.

Autoflowering *Cannabis* produce special chemicals which are most probably the reasons you are growing the plant. Psychoactivity, medicinal qualities, flavor, and smell are as important to Autoflowering *Cannabis* harvests as taste is to a harvest of ripe tomatoes. These are covered.

Next is a look at the supplies needed to grow Autoflowering *Cannabis* at home. We are not doing a commercial grow. Most of the stuff can be collected from things you already use, but Autoflowers may need some special things you don't already have.

This is followed by how to specifically grow Autoflowering *Cannabis* plants. And, once you do, how and when to harvest, cure, and store your harvest.

After an introduction to breeding your own Autoflowering *Cannabis* (remember, this is a very simple guide), I cover some of the Landrace and special strains which are the basis of most seed you can purchase today. This is capped off by some predictions for the future development of this brand-new category of hobby plants.

2

A BIT OF BOTANY AND CHEMISTRY TO GET YOU STARTED

YOU ARE A GARDENER, so you already know quite a bit about growing Autoflowering *Cannabis*. This is because all of the botanical principles that apply to growing other plants apply to Autoflowering *Cannabis* as well. The process and methods for growing a tomato are the same for growing Autoflowering *Cannabis*.

However, there is some special information that applies to growing Autoflowering *Cannabis* in particular, just as there is with growing any plant. For example, tomatoes are especially susceptible to tobacco mosaic disease. What are the equivalent, unique things you should know about growing Autoflowering *Cannabis* plants?

This requires a brief discussion of some botanical facts, specific to Autoflowering *Cannabis,* which will help you to understand how best to grow them. It is also necessary to learn something about the chemicals Autoflowering *Cannabis* produces.

LEAVES

Cannabis has a very distinctive, no doubt familiar, leaf. Each consists of a number of serrated leaflets. The first leaf pair has single, fingered leaflets. Successive leaves add leaflets with up to as many as 13 making up one leaf. Notably, as *Cannabis* plants mature, the number of leaflets on leaves at the top of the plant diminishes until the very top displays leaves of a single leaflet again.

Leaves can tell you a lot about an Autoflowering *Cannabis* plant. They can be used as a general indicator of the health of your plants, just as do the leaves of tomatoes. They should be a healthy green, though it is normal for Autoflowering *Cannabis* plants to be just a tad on the dull side, as they use everything produced in their leaves so quickly.

If leaves exhibit colors that are not green, there are many gardening books on nutrient deficiencies. While there are actually a hundred possible reason why a plant leaf displays a particular symptom, visual leaf symptoms, though far from perfect, are still useful in helping to determine nutrient deficiencies. Of course, tomato growers are big followers of leaf symptoms, and books that cover those should also be useful to the Autoflowering *Cannabis* gardener.

Autoflowering *Cannabis* leaves are naturally susceptible to problems associated with humidity. There is a thin envelope of air that surrounds all plant leaves called the boundary layer. If thick enough, this layer becomes an impediment to the release from leaves of water molecules produced during photosynthesis. In addition, CO_2 headed into the plant via stomata has problems.

As a result, the plant does not take up as much water as normal, resulting in a reduction of nutrients going into the plant. Photosynthesis may not be as efficient as it should be, because of CO_2 delivery problems. The plant is weakened. It is bad enough to have this happen to a regular plant, but Autoflowering *Cannabis* plants grow so fast, they cannot afford to miss a day recovering.

Then, there is the disease problem caused by higher humidity around leaves. The boundary layer makes a mini environment, perfect for powdery mildew spores to take hold and germinate and then dig into the leaves. And spread.

The take-home points here: when growing Autoflowering *Cannabis*, air movement is critical; in addition, it is critical to make sure your soil has all the nutrients your plants will need, so they don't develop problems.

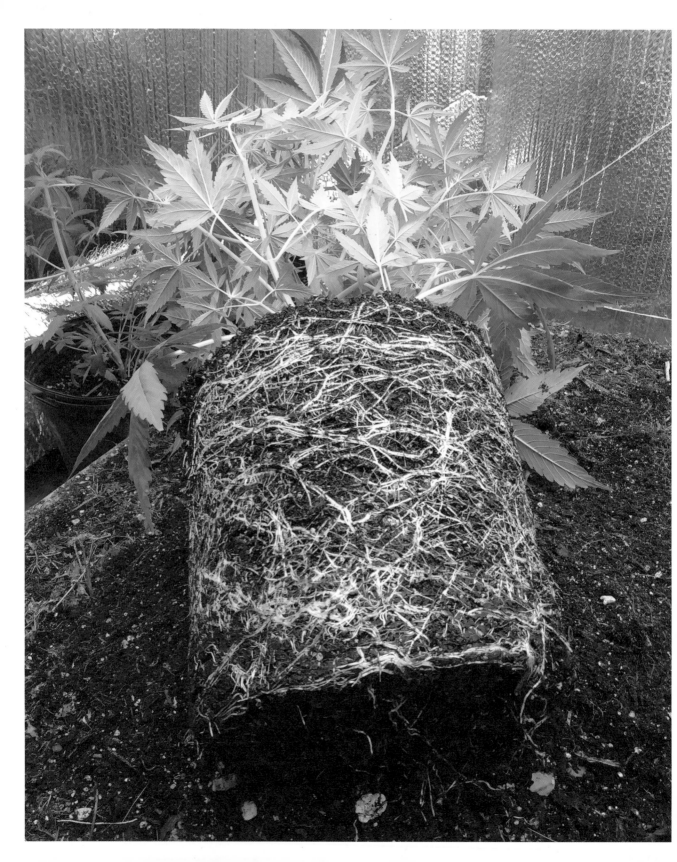

ROOTS

As all gardeners know, roots not only support the plant, they are the entry way for nutrients. Autoflowering *Cannabis* plants have a primary root with many secondary roots splaying off it. These secondary roots, in turn, branch several more times, and their growing tips are covered in root hairs.

Autoflowering *Cannabis* roots grow extremely fast, and plants can quickly become root-bound. A tomato can recover from being root-bound, but the superfast-growing Autoflowering *Cannabis* plant suffers too big a loss. It can take a week for a newly transplanted plant of any kind to return to normal growth. Due to the Autoflower's short life span, the missed time recovering can't be made up.

The takeaway from this is that Autoflowering *Cannabis* plants need ample room to grow. Their roots should not be disturbed at all. *Ever.* This means you should not attempt to transplant Autoflowering *Cannabis* seedlings, at least until after you grow a few crops to learn just how quickly they develop their root system.

MYCORRHIZAE

Almost all plants send out signals from their roots to attract specific mycorrhizal fungal types. These fungi share phosphorous, nitrogen, zinc, copper, iron, calcium, magnesium, and manganese with the plant in return for carbon-laced exudates. They are much smaller than root hairs and can mine areas of the soil that are not otherwise readily accessible to the plants' roots.

There is one particular species of mycorrhizal fungus, *Rhizophagus intraradices,* which forms this symbiotic relationship with any kind of *Cannabis,* and Autoflowering *Cannabis* is no exception. It is best to have this fungus, or at least its spores, in the soil.

In addition to the potential for bigger plants as a result of better nutrient uptake, *Rhizophagus intraradices* has the potential to help your plants fight disease, because well-fed plants remain healthy. And its presence even helps roots ward off damaging nematodes

◀ Autoflowering *Cannabis* roots grow extremely fast. Plants can become rootbound very quickly. Don't let it happen. FREHNER SEBRING

The mycorrhizal fungus which partners with Autoflowering *Cannabis* has undergone a number of name changes as a result of reclassification. It is properly called *Rhizophagus intraradices.* However, you may still find older nomenclature in use on labels. *Glomus intraradices, G. mossae, G. gregator,* and *G. etunicatum* are all the same fungus.

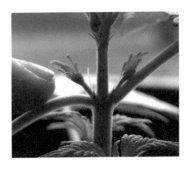

▲ Nodes along an Autoflowering *Cannabis* stem. It's a girl! Note the thin white thread, a stigma. JUDITH HOERSTING.

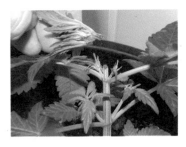

▲ Pinching just above nodes results in the development of new branches, each of which will, in turn, develop flowers. Note the tiny hairs, actually stigma, indicating the plant is a female. JUDITH HOERSTING.

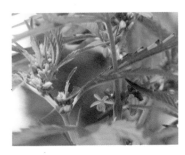

▲ Male flowers about to open and release pollen. BY THAYNE TUASON, WIKICOMMONS.

because (as with all fungi) its walls contain chitin, which root nematodes do not like.

The takeaway? *Rhizophagus intraradices* mycorrhizal fungus inoculants are now available commercially. The very same products can and should be used on tomatoes, so more and more nurseries carry it. Grow stores have many different offerings.

It is important to note that all mycorrhizal fungi do best in an organic system. In fact, ensuring that you have mycorrhizal fungi associate with your plants is a primary reason to grow organically.

NODES

Along the stems of Autoflowering *Cannabis* are nodes, areas where new branches develop. The area along the stem between these nodes is, unsurprisingly, called the inter-nodal zone. Tomato plants form stem nodes, too. It is from these nodes that tomato suckers and flower branches start to grow.

Stem nodes are the sites of undifferentiated cells, called meristem. The meristem at the growing (apical or top) tip of the plant produces the plant hormone auxin, and the presence of enough auxin at lower lateral node tips inhibits branching. Pinch a growing tip of a young Autoflowering *Cannabis* plant and you cut off the auxin supply that was keeping things in check. The meristem then develops not one but two new tips. If these, in turn, are pinched, the supply of auxins is again diminished, and two more tips grow below each new pinch.

At some point, plants lose the ability to produce new branches. Instead, a chemical is produced that converts the meristem into flower cells. Then flower buds form instead of growing tips. If you pinch at this point, you lose the flower. Unlike before, you don't get two new ones.

Whether to pinch an Autoflowering *Cannabis* is directly related to the plant's genetics. Some have been bred to produce the largest possible amount of branches and flowers. These types of

Autoflowering *Cannabis* plants lose too much valuable time when they are pinched and then they don't produce as well.

Why are nodes important, then? The home gardener is usually limited, either by space and time or by governmental fiat, in the number of plants that can be grown. Each new growing tip produced represents a potential flower source, so it is important to know if you can pinch your plant back.

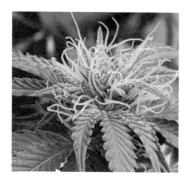

▲ Female flowers developing at the tips of branches. JUDITH HOERSTING.

AUTOFLOWERING *CANNABIS* FLOWERS

Autoflowering *Cannabis* has male and female flowers on respective plants. This is a big difference between tomatoes and Autoflowers. It is the female flowers that are prized (unless you are into breeding your own seed) because these produce the wanted chemicals. Male flowers do not. Unless a gardener wants to breed Autoflowering *Cannabis*, male plants are discarded.

Cannabis flowers, known as buds in the trade, are, botanically speaking, inflorescences of florets. A floret is just a small flower—think of what broccoli or cauliflower heads are made up of. Autoflowering *Cannabis* inflorescences are florets closely lined up on a stem or in a tight bunch.

Early in an Autoflowering *Cannabis* plant's life, close examination of what is happening at node junctions will reveal the sex of the plant long before flowering occurs. Female plants display fine filament pistils (more on pistils and stigma below), whereas tiny sacs indict male plants.

Female flowers

A female *Cannabis* floret forms a calyx. This is a single sepal that wraps itself around the female reproductive parts to protect them. In addition to holding the flower's pistils, this is where most of the plant's chemicals are produced.

The pistil, in turn, consists of an ovary, a style, and a stigma. It is sticky and holds pollen during fertilization. Tiny hairs grow out of the pistil. These are stigma, and they, too, can collect pollen.

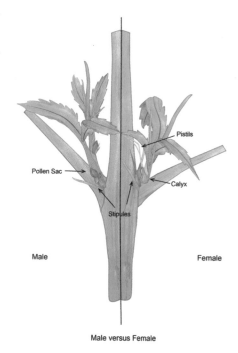

Male Female

Male versus Female

▲ Male and female flowers developing at nodes show the sex of the plant early. WINNIE CASACOP.

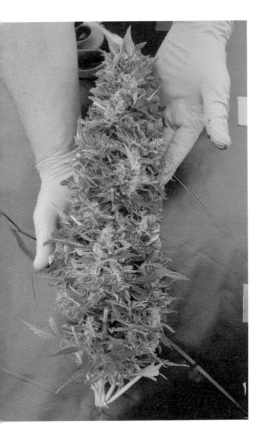

This huge cola from a New Breed Seed Autoflowering *Cannabis* plant, Timberline, VAR, is something to strive for. HAROLD FRAZIER, NEW BREED SEED.

The presence of pistils on female flowers makes it easy to distinguish a female plant from a male one—males don't have them. Stigma start out clear, or white, but as the flowers become ripe, they turn brown.

Calyxes can display all manner of color: green, yellow, pink, purple, and more depending on climate and strain. When Autoflowering *Cannabis* is grown properly, they crowd together forming what the untrained eye might call a single flower. Actually, this cluster of calyxes is known as a cola.

Calyxes make it easier for the female plant to catch the wind-borne male pollen. Most important, calyxes are covered with special glands called trichomes. These are where the desired chemicals for which the plant is grown are produced.

Each branch along a stem has the potential to develop into a cola of varying size. The top tip branch usually produces the main biggest cola, with smaller ones being produced from lower branches. Cola size is dependent on how many florets form. (Again, think of the whole cauliflower or broccoli head.)

Feminization of seeds to ensure only female plants

Since only sterile female flowers count, someone figured out how to ensure seeds would produce female plants. This can be done by rhodelization (stressing) which causes a female plant to develop a few male flowers with pollen sacs, along with female flowers. If the plant self-fertilizes, or if the pollen from this female plant is used to fertilize another female plant, then the resultant seed will produce only female plants. Using these seeds means you don't have to grow, identify, and discard male plants, and that will save you time and effort.

But the most common method to feminize seed is to use colloidal silver or gibberellic acid. Application of either to plants at the right time (for 4 weeks after lights are at 12 hours for *Cannabis indica* and *Cannabis sativa,* if you must know) causes the plant to produce flowers that contain some pollen sacs. These sacs can be removed, stored,

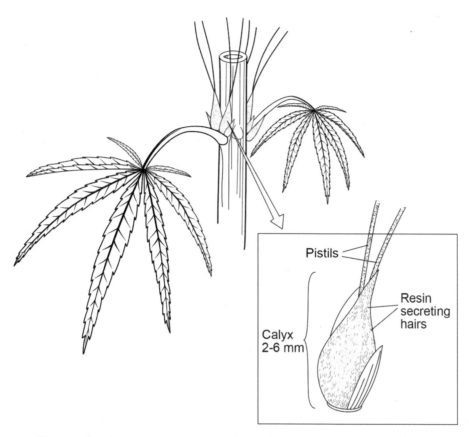

The parts of a calyx. WINNI CASACOP.

and later used to pollinate a female plant that has had flowers for 2 or 3 weeks. It takes about 6 weeks after pollination for *Cannabis indica* and *Cannabis sativa* to become ripe with seeds.

Autoflowering *Cannabis* is no different from other forms of *Cannabis*, so it is certainly possible to chemically induce rhodelization. The problem in this case is the timing because the plants grow so fast. Generally, however, if you apply one of these chemicals to forming buds, you can induce the production of pollen sacs.

Both colloidal silver as well as gibberellic acid are available on the market. You can even make your own colloidal silver. Feminization of seed is an advanced aspect of growing Autoflowering

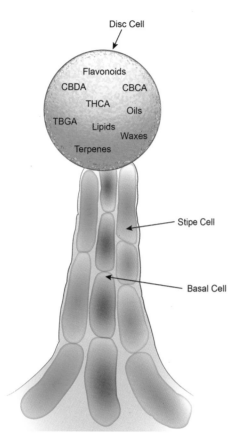

Disc Cell

Flavonoids

CBDA   CBCA

THCA

TBGA   Oils

Lipids

Waxes

Terpenes

Stipe Cell

Basal Cell

Glandular Trichome

▲ Diagram of glandular trichome. WINNIE CASACOP.

Cannabis, the details of which can be gleaned off the Internet. It is certainly not something a gardener should try to tackle for the first few grows, or probably ever.

Feminizing your own seeds might be fun as you become more and more enamored with growing Autoflowering *Cannabis.* You may decide to add this skill to your wheelbarrow and give it a try if you decide to breed your own varieties. Again, this is why Autoflowering *Cannabis* is a great hobby plant.

Fortunately, you can now buy fantastic feminized seeds from several outlets. Not only will you have less work, but the breeder provides the necessary cultural information to make your job easier, as well as producing seeds with superior genetics. This really is an easy plant to grow, but all the information you can gather helps.

Male flowers

Male Autoflowering *Cannabis* flowers have stamens and anthers that contain pollen sacs and filaments to hold the pollen sacs onto the plant. The sacs are about 5 mm (0.2 in.) in size. The most important difference between male and female Autoflowering *Cannabis* flowers, however, is that male flowers do not produce chemicals which are psychoactive. Every now and then a male plant appears. This is why you need to know what they look like.

In addition, male plants need to be removed from the growing area so that they don't pollinate females. Without males to pollinate, the female plants produce sterile flowers, known as sinsemilla.

Sometimes a female Autoflowering *Cannabis* plant develops some male flowers and *vise versa.* Plants with *both* male and female flowers on the same plant are monoecious. (They are often referred to as hermaphrodites, but this term properly refers to plants that have both male and female parts in the *same* flower.) This trait is important because it allows interested gardeners to try breeding their own varieties, adding an extra dimension to the hobby.

TRICHOMES

Autoflowering *Cannabis* produce special hair-like glands known as trichomes. These are very similar to those that cover the stems and leaves of tomatoes. In Autoflowering *Cannabis*, trichomes probably protect the plant. The substances they produce may prevent grazing by mammals and insects. In addition, they provide plant surfaces with shade protection from damaging UV waves.

Capitate stalked trichomes

If you look closely at a mature Autoflowering *Cannabis* flower (and leaves as well), you will see lots of small mushroom-like structures, 50 to 100 micrometers (0.002 to 0.004 in.) long. These are glandular trichomes.

Looking through a hand lens (or the magnification setting on your cell phone) reveals that each consists of an elongated base which holds a round head that is covered with a waxy cuticle. The setup looks like a golf ball on a tee.

Of prime importance, the synthesis of the cannabinoids and terpenoids takes place inside these trichome heads. These factories, however, are very delicate and rupture when treated roughly. Such treatment exposes the chemicals inside, which then oxidize and degrade.

Autoflower trichomes respond to improper treatment in a negative way. Physical manipulation, passage of time, and exposure to heat, air, and light are detrimental. It is critical to limit contact with glandular trichomes and to make sure plants are grown in the proper environment, and stored in one as well.

Of equal importance, the color of capitate-stalked trichomes is a great visual indicator to monitor a plant's stage of growth. In fact, the gardener can really only tell if plants are ready for harvest by tracking trichome color changes from clear to cloudy, and then to amber.

At the base of each female *Cannabis* flower is a tiny structure known as a bract, a pseudo leaf. (It is the bracts on poinsettias that give those plants their color.) This bract helps hold the flower

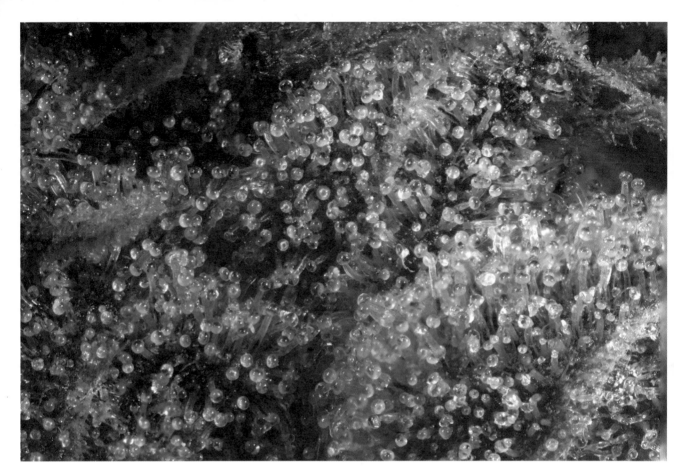

▲ Autoflowering *Cannabis* trichome under magnification. Note that some are clear, some are cloudy, and others are amber. FRED GUNNERSON, SOFRESH FARMS.

together. As important (and maybe even more so), these bracts are covered with capitate-stalked trichomes.

When you have the right genetics and do a good job helping these plants grow, glandular trichomes form a dense coating that is known as sugar or frost. This a is very desirable trait and production of plants with lots and lots of trichomes is your goal.

Bulbous and capitate sessile trichomes

There are two kinds of smaller trichomes. These cover male plants, which do not produce many glandular trichomes (alas). The first are known as bulbous trichomes, which are only 10 to 15 micrometers

(0.0004 to 0.0006 in.), making them the smallest of the trichomes. They cover the entire plant.

The last group are the capitate sessile trichomes. These have a stalk and a head just like the capitate stalked trichomes, but don't produce the same amount or kinds of resins as do the bigger bulbous glands. They also cover the plant, being even more abundant than the bulbous types.

A SUMMARY OF WHAT TO EXPECT AS AN AUTOFLOWERING *CANNABIS* PLANT GROWS

O.K. Now you know enough of the plant parts to follow the growth pattern of Autoflowering *Cannabis* as the plant goes through various stages of its growth.

First the seeds soak up water and germinate, in sometimes as little as 30 hours. Seed cotyledons unfurl and are followed by the seedling stage during which the plant develops 2 embryonic leaves and then between 4 and 8 more mature leaves of increasing size. Depending on the environmental conditions, this stage can last from 1 to 3 weeks.

The vegetative or growth stage is next. The stem grows thicker and taller, and side nodes develop. More leaves are produced and new branches too. The vegetative stage lasts up to 5 months in a *Cannabis indica* or *Cannabis sativa*. Autoflowering plants can move out of the vegetative stage after only 3 short weeks.

Next is the pre-flowering stage. The plant continues to grow. The male plants display a small, green sac-like structure at nodes. (This sac will eventually fill with pollen.) White hairs, the pistils of female plants, form at the nodes of female plants. Pistils are distinct female plant organs that consist of an ovary, a style, and a sticky stigma which is where male pollen is first collected. It is the color of the stigma which helps determine ripeness. Because of this importance, the term stigma is often used to refer to the entire pistil.

The flowering stage occurs after these early sex precursors develop more. Buds form and start to grow. Trichomes become visible, coating bracts, flowers, and nearby leaves, causing them to them to get sticky. The plant may also develop an odor characteristic of the variety being grown. This odor is from the chemicals produced in trichomes. Male pollen sacs (if male plants are allowed to remain) fill and open, spilling pollen.

When the pistils on flowers turn from white to rusty brown, it is a signal that the plants are ripening and nearing the harvest stage. This often starts with the top buds of the main cola and moves down to lower colas during the course of a week or so.

The glandular trichomes gradually turn from clear to opaque. On average, once 20 to 50% of them are milky in appearance, it is time to start the harvest. After trichomes become cloudy, they turn amber or honey-colored. Time to harvest for sure. The pistils turn brown and dry.

The Autoflowering *Cannabis* harvest stage can occur after an astonishingly brief 5 or 6 weeks (though usually it is 8 weeks or a bit longer). After it is finished, the harvest will require collecting, drying, and curing. Drying can take about a week or so. Curing is an ongoing process that can take place as the Autoflowering *Cannabis* is stored.

SOME *CANNABIS* CHEMISTRY TO KNOW

Traditionally, *Cannabis* was grown for making rope, producing cloth, and making paper. I don't wish to delude anyone, however. It is the chemicals in *Cannabis* that today make Autoflowering *Cannabis* of interest to the home gardener.

These chemicals cause the psychoactive highs and impart the medical effects for which many forms of *Cannabis* are known. I use the plural because different chemical mixes in different varieties of *Cannabis* plants cause varying degrees and types of psychoactivity or impact different parts of the body in different ways. Chemicals that don't produce psychoactive effects may impact other aspects of our psychology and physiology, causing calming, reduction of inflammation, prevention of certain kinds of seizures, and more.

CANNABINOIDS

There are all sorts of numbers tossed about as to how many different chemical compounds are produced by a *Cannabis* plant. Suffice to note there are over 100 that react chemically with receptors found in both plants and animals. You will have heard of some of these cannabinoids, at least in their abbreviated form, as they include THC (tetrahydrocannabinol), CBD (cannabidiol), and CBN (cannabinol).

Actually, cannabinoids are in acid form inside the Autoflowering *Cannabis* plant, so they are more properly named THCA (tetrahydrocannabinol acid), CBDA (cannabidiol acid), and CBNA (cannabinol acid). In these acidic forms, cannabinoids are not bioavailable and humans cannot react to them. They cannot be absorbed. We will stick with the non-acid abbreviations in this text.

It is drying and, in particular, heating that converts these chemical compounds from acids to their absorbable form. This is via a process known as decarboxylation. Scientifically, a cannabinoid gives up a single carbon dioxide molecule. If you skip decarboxylation, your Autoflowering *Cannabis* might just as well be lettuce insofar as psychoactive or medical activity is concerned.

Once decarboxylated, however, cannabinoids can be absorbed and will react with the human body. A lot of studies are being conducted to figure out just exactly what these impacts are and how they happen. (Stay tuned.)

How cannabinoids work

Many functions in the human body such as sleep, mood, pain, immune system responses, hunger, and memory are regulated by a messaging chain, the endocannabinoid system. The chemicals used in this regulation are endocannabinoids. They attach to special receptors mostly concentrated in the nervous system, brain, immune system, and organs.

When cannabinoids from any *Cannabis* plant are present, they work with the body's endocannabinoid receptors to produce a variety of effects. These receptors are sensitive to cannabinoids, which interfere with or change the body's natural chemical messages.

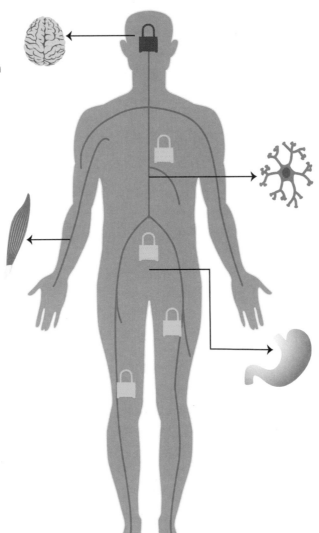

Brain
- Cannabidiol reduces seizures in Dravet's syndrome, a rare form of epilepsy.
- Cannabis is effective against nausea.

Central Nervous System
- Cannabis taken in various forms has been shown to reduce chronic pain.

Muscle
- Adults with multiple sclerosis have fewer muscle spasms.

Gut
- Patients with inflammatory bowel disease report improvement after smoking cannabis.

 CB$_1$

CB$_1$ receptors are concentrated in the brain and regulate areas involved with mood, memory, appetite, and movement.

 CB$_2$

CB$_2$ receptors are mostly found in muscles, bones, the liver, and the immune system. When triggered, they tend to have beneficial effects, like toning down inflammation.

Only the endocannabinoid receptors found in the brain react to THC producing psychoactive effects. There is a second set of receptors which are all located outside the brain and are not involved in psychoactivity, but are responsible for a number of other physiological responses such as inflammation and pain. These react to CBD.

In sum, when an individual ingests *Cannabis*, the endocannabinoid system becomes overloaded as THC and the other phytocannabinoids from the plant attach to receptors all through the body. This interferes with the activity of the body's natural endocannabinoids. And, because the endocannabinoid system is distributed throughout the body, the impacts can be wide-ranging.

PSYCHOACTIVE CANNABINOIDS

To keep things simple, the Autoflowering *Cannabis* gardener only needs to be aware of a few cannabinoids. Incidentally, these are all odor free. However, their presence or lack thereof helps define how Autoflowering *Cannabis* impacts the body. Let's explore them.

THC

The main psychoactive cannabinoid is delta-9-tetrahydrocannabinoid acid, THC. This is the primary cannabinoid produced by the psychoactive varieties of *Cannabis*. This is what imparts the characteristics of a "high."

THC attaches itself to endocannabinoid receptors in the brain causing psychoactivity. Initially, these reactions to THC can also increase heartbeat, cause anxiety, or sedate. There is a diminution of the psychoactive effects at high (sorry) doses. This is because the body's receptors become saturated. Signals are blocked by other cannabinoids.

Usually, ingesting too much THC is not a problem. However, it can cause bloodshot eyes and dry mouth. It can also be responsible for any anxiety attacks, short-term memory loss, dizziness, or even nausea.

◀ Endocannabinoid guide. WINNI CASACOP.

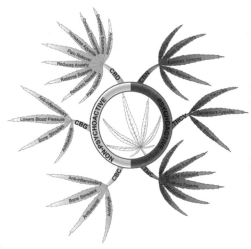

Cannabinoids are the group of chemical compounds found in the cannabis plant that have physical and mental effects when they interact with cannabinoid receptors in your cells.

Cannabinoid Guide

▲ Cannabinoid guide. WINNI CASACOP.

Cannabis is often recommended to chemotherapy patients to control nausea. It is the THC that does this. The pain relief prescription drugs Cesamet and Marinol provide relief because of THC they contain.

Breeders have been able to achieve remarkably high (again, sorry, but this is exactly the right word!) THC percentages that can equal over 30% of the plant's dry weight. This is a huge amount, much more than is found in plants growing in nature. Each gardener will have different tolerances to using them. Until you understand their impact, remember the Goldilocks Rule: use in moderation.

THCV

Tetrahydrocannabivarin (whew, no wonder you don't hear about this one), THCV, is a different form of THC that has different impacts on the endocannabinoid system. There is not a lot of research, however, on these cannabinoids, though there are some studies on its ability to help with certain forms of glucose intolerance.

CBN

CBN, for cannabinol, is found in Autoflowering *Cannabis*. It is a by-product of degradation of THC. It usually doesn't exist in large quantities in fresh plants.

CBN is psychoactive and has sedating properties. It is considered an anti-psychotic by some. Studies show varying impacts on such diverse human (and pet) aliments as diabetes, cancer, neurodegenerative diseases, Crohn's, and inflammation.

NON-PSYCHOACTIVE CANNABINOIDS

There are lots of non-psychoactive cannabinoids. These impact only endocannabinoid nodes in the body, not in the brain. As a result of a tremendous amount of publicity in the first part of this century (a news story of their impact on a child's severe seizures that appeared on national TV in the United States and Canada), they became almost as popularly known as THC. There is no reason a home gardener can't grow their own.

CBD

Cannabidiolic acid converts to CBD, the number two cannabinoid in Autoflowering *Cannabis*, constituting up to 40% of the cannabinoids in a plant's resin. It interacts with a much broader range of endocannabinoid receptors than THC (but does not react with the receptors that THC does). This is the chemical touted for its impact on certain forms of epilepsy, but it has a wide range of impacts on the human body.

CBD has been found to actually interfere with the intensity of THC. It is being studied for its impact on anxiety, depression, and pediatric epilepsy. It is antibacterial and has been studied in light of positive responses to dealing with MRSA-type pathogens.

In addition, CBD reduces pain and inflammation. It has become very popular as a home remedy for muscle pains and as a sleep aid. One of the most promising attributes appears to be the ability to aid in protecting the brain after an injury such as a concussion. Clearly, the research has just begun, and no doubt more uses will be discovered for CBD.

CBG

In terms of percentages, after THC and CBD comes cannabigerol or CBG. It is actually the precursor of THC and CBD and is converted to the other two by cellular enzymatic activity.

CBG has gained attention of late because mouse studies show it is effective in helping with irritable bowel diseases. It is strongly antibacterial and antifungal and is being studied as an anti-tumor agent and as an aid in treating prostate diseases.

CBG can interact with cellular systems in addition to the endocannabinoid. Only about 1 percent of the cannabinoids are in this group, though this can be increased by breeding, as can the other cannabinoids.

▶ Terpenes' major benefits.

CBC

Cannabichromene (again, you can see why abbreviations are used), CBC, is only found in some Autoflowering *Cannabis* plants. It isn't psychoactive, but it is a moderator of pain. CBC has antibacterial and antifungal properties and has been shown to reduce acne.

TERPENES

In addition to cannabinoids, over 200 chemicals called terpenes have been found in *Cannabis* thus far. Terpenes and their oxidized forms, terpenoids, are odoriferous compounds produced by all plants and animals. Each has a unique smell, taste, and effects. They serve a number of functions. Bacteria, for example, communicate by producing and "reading" each other's terpenes.

There are more than 30,000 terpenes found in nature. The exact same terpene can be made by different plants: lemon, lime, and orange trees, for example. Still, many terpenes produced by *Cannabis* cannot be found in other plants.

Terpenes give Autoflowering *Cannabis* plants their characteristic smells and flavors. They bind to the cannabinoid receptors in the brain and body where they chemically complement THC. Autoflowering *Cannabis* would not be the same without them since they blend with (odorless) cannabinoids. Think of the smells of lemon, orange, or pine, as all of these scents and flavors are due to terpenes.

While there is only one kind of THC, there are lots of kinds of terpenes. The way *Cannabis* affects you, therefore, depends an awful lot on the mix of terpenes (and other cannabinoids) present. Some are noted for imparting pain relief, others for reducing inflammation, inducing sleep, reducing anxiety, providing focus, or serving as anti-microbial agents. Each terpene imparts a different feeling to the experience of using *Cannabis*, and knowing their mix, or "profile," in a plant can define the experience before one ingests.

The same variety of *Cannabis* grown under different conditions can show a different profile. This has led to a confusing array of

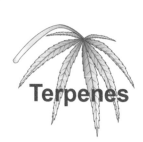

Terpenes

Myrcene

Benefits
Analgesic
Antibacterial
Antidiabetic
Anti-insomnia
Antiproliferative
Anti-inflammatory
Antimutagenic
Antipsychotic
Antispasmodic

Sources
Cannabis
West Indian
  Bay Tree
Houttuynia
Lemon grass
Mango
Myrcia
Thyme
Verbena
Cardamom
Hops

Pinene

Benefits
Analgesic
Antibacterial
Antioxidant
Antiproliferative
Anti-inflammatory

Sources
Cannabis
Makrut lime
  fruit
Turpentine tree
Juniper berries
Ironwort
Pine resin
Pine nuts
Conifers
Sage

Humulene

Benefits
Analgesic
Antibacterial
Anorectic
Antiproliferative
Anti-inflammatory

Sources
Cannabis
Vietnamese
  coriander
Japanese
  spicebush
Common sage
Pine trees
Oranges
Ginseng
Spearmint
Ginger
Hops

Limonene

Benefits
Analgesic
Antidepressant
Antifungal
Antiproliferative
Anti-inflammatory
Immunostimulant
Gastroesophageal
  reflux

Sources
Cannabis
Oranges
Lemons
Celery
Dill
Fennel
Lime
Nutmeg
Rosemary

Caryophyllene

Benefits
Analgesic
Antidepressant
Antifungal
Antiproliferative
Anti-inflammatory
Neuroprotective
Antioxidant
Anxiolytic

Sources
Cannabis
Black caraway
Oregano
Black pepper
Lavender
Ylang-ylang
Cloves
Hops
Rosemary
Basil

Terpinolene

Benefits
Antibacterial
Anti-insomnia
Antifungal
Antiproliferative
Antioxidant

Sources
Cannabis
Cedarwood
Grapefruit
Marjoram
Apricot
Nutmeg
Oregano
Papaya
Parsley
Sage

Linalool

Benefits
Analgesic
Antidepressant
Sedative
Antipsychotic
Anti-inflammatory
Anti-epileptic

Sources
Cannabis
Lavender
Basil
Hops
Goldenrods
Indian bay leaf
Mint
Laurels
Cinnamon
Rosewood

Eucalyptol

Benefits
Analgesic
Antibacterial
Antidiabetic
Antipsychotic
Anti-inflammatory
Antispasmodic
Anti-insomnia
Antiproliferative
Antimutagenic

Sources
Cannabis
Eucalyptus
Blueberry
Camphor laurel
Bay leaves
Tea tree
Sweet basil
Wormwood
Rosemary
Common sage

Borneol

Benefits
Analgesic
Antibacterial
Antidiabetic
Antipsychotic
Anti-inflammatory
Antispasmodic
Anti-insomnia
Antiproliferative
Antimutagenic

Sources
Cannabis
Cardamom
Coriander
Camphor
Marjoram
Pine needle
Saffron
Rosemary
Turmeric

names which has complicated breeding and buying *Cannabis*. They are often, incidentally, as useless as are the names of tomato varieties.

The different mixes of cannabinoids and terpenes is what makes growing, and actually harvesting and using your Autoflowering *Cannabis*, interesting. It is a good idea to become familiar with the major terpenes as they will help you describe your plant. Follow the smells.

SOME IMPORTANT TERPENE PROFILES

More and more commercial vendors are using a system that lists and describes the terpene content of the product. This system is rightfully replacing an *indica* versus *sativa* method of choosing which *Cannabis* to grow or use and provides a much more exact preview of what to expect.

Today, there is an ever-increasing number of studies designed to shed light on the subject. As a result, we are beginning to understand that the terpenes and terpenoids have much to do with the type of high induced by *Cannabis*. Terpenes are made up only of carbon and hydrogen so they are hydrocarbons. Terpenoids are terpenes altered by oxidation and contain other elements. Both act in synergy with cannabinoids and create an "entourage effect."

Instead of *indica* versus *sativa*, we now know that terpenoid alcohols such as linalool, bisabool, guaiol, as well as beta-myrcene are partially responsible for couch-lock and terpenes that create the *sativa*-type high include terpinolene and beta-caryophyllene. It is possible to learn to taste and recognize the smells of terpenoids and terpenes just as one does with wine.

With *Cannabis*, the ensemble effect comes into play. The sum of the impacts is greater than the individual components. Various terpenes work together better than they do alone, creating special impacts.

Borneol

This terpene smells like menthol and camphor. It is found in cinnamon, wormwood, and galanga. Borneol imparts a calming effect and can be very sedating. It is also used to repel insects. Strains of *Cannabis* that have it include Diamond Girl and Green-o-matic.

Beta caryophyllene

The only terpene to intersect directly with the endocannabinoid system, beta caryophyllene is a spicy terpene that smells somewhat like black pepper, in which it is also found. It is also found in cloves, cinnamon, oregano, basil, and rosemary, and in green leafy vegetables. Because of its complex makeup, it survives temperatures used to make extract products and so is found in lots of them. Strains with beta caryophyllene include Skywalker, Haze#2, and Super Silver Haze.

Beta caryophyllene is used as an anti-inflammatory. It is being studied to help deal with alcoholism. As a topical and ingested, it has analgesic and anti-anxiety impacts. It also gives a characteristic odor when oxidized, and it is said this is the scent that law enforcement drug dogs were trained to locate.

Eucalyptol

As you would expect, this terpene is what gives eucalyptus its spicy, minty smell. It is also found in tea tree, amphora, sage, and rosemary. Strains that contain eucalyptus include Chem Dawg, Bubba Kush, and King's Kush. Eucaluptol is an antibacterial used in mouthwashes and body deodorants.

Humulene

Hops, a botanical relative of Autoflowering *Cannabis*, contains lots of humulene, which has a woody, earthy smell and is found in black pepper, cloves, as well as sage. Strains with humulene include White Widow, Skywalker OG, Headband, Girl Scout Cookies, and Sour Diesel.

Humulene is an appetite suppressant. It relieves inflammation and is an antibacterial.

Limonene

Limonene is the second most abundant terpene in *Cannabis* and, as its name suggests, is found in large quantities in citrus rinds. Any strain with a citrus fruit or sour in its name contains limonene. Jack the Ripper, Lemon Skunk, Jack Herer, OG Kush, Sour Diesel, Tangerine, Super Lemon Haze, and Durban Poison are all notable strains that contain limonene.

Limonene is antifungal and antibacterial. It reduces stress and elevates moods. It is considered the terpene that imparts the energetic high associated with some *Cannabis* varieties. It is being studied as it appears to kill cancer cells in lab tests.

Linalool

This terpene imparts a spicy, flowery smell. It is found in lavender, mint, cinnamon, and coriander. Strains that contain linalool include Amnesia Haze, Grape Ape, G-13, Lavender, LA Confidential, and OG Shark.

Linalool is very relaxing and sedative in its effects. Some use it in oil form for treatment of burns and acne. It is said to help with arthritis, insomnia, seizures, and depression.

Myrcene

Myrcene has an earthy, musky smell, which is also found in hops. Some suggest it resembles the smell of cloves. This is the terpene that imparts the characteristic underlying smell of Cannabis, probably because it is the dominate terpene in *Cannabis*. In some strains, 60 to 65 percent of the terpenes are myrcene.

Strains that have high amounts of myrcene are sedative in effects. Look for it in Skunk, White Widow, White Rhino, and Mango. Many associate the couch-lock feeling with *Cannabis indica* because it accompanies the use of many *Cannabis indica* varieties. Actually, it is the myrcene in *Cannabis* that induces this feeling.

Pinene

There are two types of pinene terpenes in *Cannabis,* alpha and beta pinenes. Both smell like pine needles, in which you can of course find it. You can also find pinene in rosemary, basil, and parsley. Strains that contain pinene include Super Silver Haze, Train Wreck, Cheese, Bubba Kush, Dutch Treat, Jack Herer, Strawberry Cough, Blue Dream, and Romulan.

Pinene is a solvent that breaks down plastics, and it is one of the reasons *Cannabis* should be stored in glass jars rather than plastic containers. Pinene helps with asthma. It is anti-inflammatory and helps with arthritis.

Terpineol

While the name suggests turpentine smell, terpineol actually imparts a lilac or apple blossom odor. It is used in perfumes and flavorings.

OG Kush, Girl Scout Cookies, White Rhino, and Jack Herer strains contain significant amounts of terpineol. Terpineol induces a very relaxed mood, often described as couch-lock. In addition to being a relaxing agent, it is said to have anti-oxidant properties.

Replacement of the *sativa* versus *indica* classification

Traditionally, people grew and selected *Cannabis* for consumption based on its classification as either a *sativa* or an *indica* plant. The former was said to induce an uplifting and energizing high, while the latter was noted for inducing lethargy and deep relaxation.

Terpenes, however, represent a much more accurate measure of the potential impacts of ingesting *Cannabis* and are more probably the cause of the effects felt. There is growing evidence that terpenes have quite a bit to do with the different types of effects caused by ingesting *Cannabis.* THC, CBD, etc. have predictable impacts, but these impacts are altered depending on the accompanying terpene mix. Myrcene, linalool, and nerolidol create a sedative high, while pinene or limonene mixes leave the user feeling much more energetic.

FLAVONOIDS PROVIDE COLOR
AND ADD TO TASTE AND SMELL

There is a third set of compounds in Autoflowering *Cannabis* that need to be highlighted. These are "flavonoids," compounds responsible for some of the taste and smell of Autoflowering *Cannabis* and also for the non-green pigments found in vegetables and fruits. They protect the plants from UV rays and deter pests, both grazers and disease-causers.

Flavonoids exist elsewhere in the plant kingdom with over 6,000 identified. About 20 of these are in Autoflowering *Cannabis*. (Some of these flavonoids are unique to *Cannabis* plants.) This represents about 10% of the chemical compound mix in these plants, so they are not insignificant. They are thought to modulate the effects of THC.

Flavonoids are also responsible for giving leaves and flowers their colors. They are visible when not masked by green chlorophyll. In addition to imparting color to *Cannabis*, flavonoids create odor and flavor and react with cannabinoids in synergistic ways.

Anthocyanins

Anthocyanins are plant chemicals that cause the red, blues, and purples of grapes, cherries, and blueberries. They are found in Autoflowering *Cannabis*, where reds are expressed when the soil is acidic and purples as the soil becomes neutral. At some point as the pH becomes more alkaline (goes up), these colors disappear because the anthocyanins break apart. You don't always see anthocyanins because of the presence of over-riding green chlorophyll molecules.

Cannaflavin A and B

Cannaflavin A and B are strong anti-inflammatory agents. So far, they have only been found in *Cannabis*. One study found cannaflavin A to be more effective than aspirin as an anti-inflammatory.

Beta-sitosterol

Beta-sitosterol is found in avocados and nuts. It is an anti-inflammatory.

Vitexin and isovitexi

These two flavonoids were studied and shown to have anti-cancer effects, one paper suggesting that they prevent cancer by causing cancer cells to degrade and die.

Apigenin

This is a highly studied flavonoid with anti-anxiety and anti-inflammatory capabilities. Several studies suggest they stop the growth of breast cancer cells.

Kaempferol

Kaempferol is being studied to treat heart problems. It is a known anti-cancer agent and has antidepressant properties.

Luteolin

Clover contains luteolin. In is antibacterial and is being studied as an anti-tumor agent.

Apigenin

This is one of the most studied of all the flavonoids. It is found in celery and parsley and chamomile tea. It appears to inhibit the growth of breast cancer and is an anti-anxiety as well as an anti-inflammatory agent.

Quercetin

This flavonoid is found in many fruits, and vegetables as well. It is also found in wines, green tea, and berries. It is considered to be an anti-cancer agent and an anti-oxidant and great for relieving pain.

Catechins

Catechins are found in cocoa and tea. They can have antioxidant properties and have shown cardiovascular benefits including helping to maintain cholesterol levels.

Orientin

Orientin is a flavonoid with vasodilator properties and is being studied for heart impacts. It is an anti-aging, anti-inflammatory, antibacterial, and painkilling flavonoid.

FUTURE STUDIES

At some point the restrictions against studying *Cannabis* will be lifted and a great deal more will be learned about all of the compounds in the plants. They have already been shown to be anti-oxidant, anti-aging, anti-viral, antibacterial, anti-inflammatory, good for vasodilation, cardio-protective, radiation protective, neuro-protective, antidepressant, anti-adipogenesis, and pain-relieving. (Wow!)

THAT IS ALL YOU NEED

This is really all the specialized knowledge you will need to grow Autoflowering *Cannabis*, maybe even a bit more than you need! Anything more complicated is beyond the scope of this book. If you want more information, however, there is plenty to be had. The Internet is your immediate source for anything upon which you want to expand.

There is an ever-expanding universe of research papers involving *Cannabis* and Autoflowering *Cannabis*. This research is important because previous laws restricted it or, as in the case of the United States, ensured studies were designed to prove the evils of *Cannabis*.

It is always a good idea to keep abreast of new studies that pertain to your hobbies. In the instance of *Cannabis*, new discoveries are being made all the time. Again, refer to the Internet, which is a great tool to help you in growing Autoflowering *Cannabis*. Let's look at other useful tools in the next chapter.

3

EQUIPMENT AND SUPPLIES YOU WILL NEED

As A GARDENER, you can appreciate that all you really need to grow any plant are seeds, soil, a container, and light. After all, how much do you need to buy to grow a pot or two of tomatoes?

Still, as with any specialty, there are some things you will need to buy. My suggestion is to get to know these plants before buying much equipment. What you have on hand, for the most part, will suffice.

Whether you buy or already own, it is important to get everything on hand before you start. You will be amazed at how fast Autoflowering *Cannabis* plants develop. You cannot afford to miss a day of good growth simply because you don't have something. If an Autoflowering *Cannabis* plant requires something, you need to supply it without delay.

SEEDS

Let's start with Autoflowering *Cannabis* seed. This is perhaps the most difficult supply to acquire. It is going to be a while before you can buy from a seed rack in a big-box store or at a local nursery. You will need to find a source for Autoflowering *Cannabis* seed until they become better known and until the impacts and stigma of prohibition end.

44 •

In Canada, and in an increasing number of the United States and several other countries around the world, *Cannabis* prohibition has ended. Finding Autoflowering *Cannabis* seed is not going to be too much of a problem. In these places, there are breeders who are allowed to sell Autoflowering *Cannabis* seeds at licensed dispensaries.

Other places to find seeds are at *Cannabis* conventions, festivals, and trade shows. These almost always include vendors who sell *Cannabis* seeds. Even so, you may have to search for Autoflowers.

And, of course, the Internet is another fertile (sorry) source for purchasing Autoflowering *Cannabis* seeds. You can locate all of the sites that sell them using any search engine. However, it is important to understand your particular government's rules regarding receiving *Cannabis* seed through the mail or other delivery services.

Finally, you might be able to trade seed with friends who also grow Autoflowering *Cannabis*. Remember that this is a plant you can breed on your own. Of course, you need seeds to start with.

Do not to skimp on seed. Spend on genetics and feminization. You get what you pay for, and in this instance, what you want to pay for is information and a lot of previous effort getting rid of susceptibility to diseases, perfecting taste and cannabinoid content, and the like.

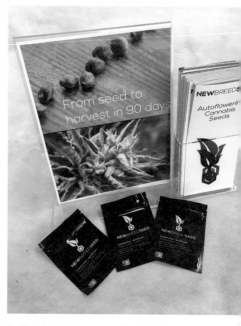

▲ Back in the 60s, no one imagined there would be *Cannabis* seed available in commercial seed packets.

Genetics

Autoflowering *Cannabis* seeds come from crosses made between diminutive *Cannabis ruderalis* plants and one or both of the larger *Cannabis* cousins. Some of the earliest successful crosses occurred in the 1970s, but not much came of these efforts. It was just too hard a to get consistency from generation to generation.

The first commercial strain of Autoflowering was (and still is) called Lowryder. A small plant, only 12 to 18 inches tall, it was the perfect size for a prohibition plant because it was great for growing in hidden-away spots, say a closet or a basement crawl space used to hide a grow.

The success of the Lowryder breeding is credited to the discovery of some Autoflowering males that became great genetic stock.

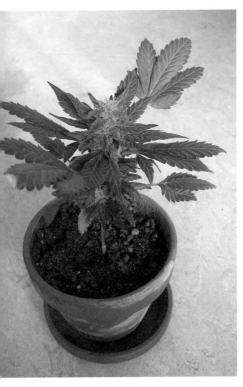

▲ A Lowryder plant, the Autoflowering variety that started it all. ERIK FENDERSON, WIKICOMMONS.

New Autoflowering *Cannabis* varieties followed, and while there are lots of existing ones from which to choose, new ones are constantly being developed. Things are constantly improving.

What to look for when you buy Autoflowering *Cannabis* seeds? The first thing is a description of the plant. How tall will it grow? What are its habit like? This will help you to determine pot size and growing location. It will also help determine if the plant needs to be pinched or not.

The most important information, however, is the number of days it takes for the seed to go from germination to harvest. Your experience will probably be slightly different from the breeder's, but you should get a very good approximation of what to expect. It had better be a very good seed if you buy it without this number.

Knowing parentage can help, too. Just be aware that more and more crosses come into the market every year. Some of these have wholly new (and often ridiculous) names. Others reveal their genetic lineage with familiar stock used in their naming.

Feminized seeds

Starting out, use feminized seeds. After all, the point of growing any *Cannabis* (unless you want to make paper or cloth) is to produce sinsemilla, females with unpollinated flowers. These produce the wanted cannabinoids and terpenoids, as you now know. Why waste time on growing males?

Autoflowering *Cannabis* breeders

In order to get feminized seeds, buy from well-known, reliable breeders. There are a few who have been improving Autoflowering *Cannabis* genetics for years and who sell only female seeds.

There are more breeders to be sure. (I list several in the appendix.) They are producing plants that have higher THC and CBD content, resist mildews and other fungal diseases, and carry other specialized and desired traits. Use the Internet to check reputations and offerings and look for new ones in your area.

Seed handling

One big difference between Autoflowering *Cannabis* seeds and those of tomatoes is that *Cannabis* seed can be pricey, especially if you are buying those that will develop new, unique varieties or those that produce exceptional crops, either in terms of chemistry or yield.

Since they cost so much, you will want to handle seeds properly. As with any seeds, the main concern is proper storage. Ideally you should keep your Autoflowering *Cannabis* seeds between 4.5 and 7.2°C (40 and 45°F). And, you should store them where there is low humidity. You can use a refrigerator, but make sure you keep the seeds in a tightly sealed container.

GROWING MEDIA

After genetics comes soil. It is really best to simply buy new soil for your first few grows. Use it and then toss it onto the compost pile after you harvest your plants. Later, once you become familiar with the needs of these plants grown under your particular conditions, you can make or mix your own designer soils.

A bit of caution must be exercised. One of the great attributes of Autoflowering *Cannabis* is that plants don't need much by way of supplemental feeding. This really makes things easy, but you must be careful. Tomato growers know that if you give a fast-growing plant too much nitrogen, for example, it won't flower properly, if at all. It just produces lots of big leaves. The ability to grow without much fuss is one of the joys of tomatoes and Autoflowering *Cannabis*.

Soil

Only use a well-draining organic soil with a pH between 6 and 6.5. Again, to accomplish this for your first grows, it is best to just buy specially designed organic soil for growing *Cannabis* from a grow store or nursery. Once you work with it and grow a few plants, you will get a feel for what you might use (or not) to make your own soils for future grows.

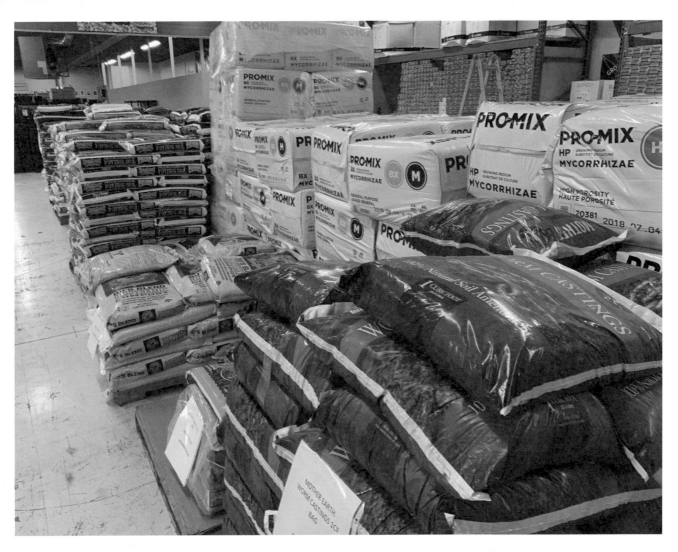

▲ For your first grows, buy soil from a grow store. JUDITH HOERSTING.

An organic soil that is good for tomatoes will be great for grow-ing Autoflowering *Cannabis*, provided it doesn't have too much fertilizer added as this makes them grow too fast and they become spindly. There are any number of commercial soils you can buy.

Do not use heavy wet bags of compost or soil. You want a light and fluffy soil mix. Ask grow stores what they recommend based on customer comments and experience. Just make sure to tell them you want an organic soil.

pH

Whatever you use, your mix should have a pH between 6 and 6.5 as this is the pH at which the soil food web operates best in feeding *Cannabis*. Home gardeners should be familiar with the chart that shows which nutrients are tied up at various soil pH levels. This chemistry really applies when it comes to Autoflowering *Cannabis*, as they grow so fast, you need things to be right all the time.

My soil mix starts with compost and vermicompost because they are teeming with soil food web life. The only microbial addition is mycorrhizal fungi (*Rhizophagus intraradices*) because compost does not support mycorrhizae.

To finish the base, add an equal amount of coir to increase organic matter and drainage. The latter is enhanced further by adding in an equal amount of perlite.

Now add nutrients. Humic acids and kelp, ¼ cup per 5 gallons of soil for fungal growth, bat guano (up to 1 cup) for bacterial food. Based on testing of nutrients and pH, add blood meal for nitrogen, rock phosphate for phosphorous, wood ash for potassium, and Epsom salt for magnesium. Crushed crab shell is great for calcium and magnesium. Dolomite lime will help balance pH and supply magnesium.

In fact, professional growers are so concerned about pH that if soil is out of range, they usually don't even try and amend it back to where they want it. They replace it instead. This is the case when growing Autoflowers. Have your soil tested or test it yourself with a pH meter or test strips before you begin. Test your water as well.

Dolomite lime, with a pH of 7, is the key to raising the pH in your soil *before* you plant. It doesn't really work fast enough once a plant is growing. Instead consider baking soda, calcium carbonate, hydrated lime, or potassium sulfate. Or, use an organic hydroponics solution designed to raise the pH.

If you need to lower the pH of your soil mix, add sulphur—again, well before you plant. It is perhaps easier to buy an organic solution designed to keep hydroponic systems in the right range. You could

It is easy to make your own super soil mix for growing Autoflowering *Cannabis*. Do it right and you won't have to fertilize your plants.

employ nitric and hydrochloric acid, but these are a bit dicey to handle. Instead, plain old lemon juice in water may be your best bet, and is the easiest to obtain.

Information is power

It always makes sense for any gardener to gather base data. This will make it possible to make corrections and adjustments if needed. Even though most gardeners don't, you should have your soil tested or do it yourself, both for nutrients and minerals as well as for its microbiology, i.e., its fungi and bacteria. (You should do the same thing for your tomato soil as well—but you probably don't!) Why not start this hobby out right by testing?

It is possible that, after you grow a crop or two, you will discover a need to add something to your soil. There are any number of places to turn to for information that matches your soil's deficiency with the proper supplement. (See, e.g., *Teaming with Nutrients: The Organic Grower's Guide to Optimizing Plant Nutrition*, Timber Press, 2013.)

Coco coir and perlite

There is a trend to grow commercial *Cannabis* using a mix that includes coconut coir and perlite. Coir is the outer husk of the coconut, and perlite is blown-up volcanic rock.

If it is good enough for commercial growing, it surely will work at home. Coir has a lot of the properties that have made peat moss popular, but coir is more sustainable. It also has higher microbiology. It holds tremendous amounts of water, so growing in it can be sort of like growing hydroponically. Because it holds so much water, aerating it is important.

This is where the perlite comes in. It is light, airy, and porous, which makes it a perfect complement to the coir. And, it will hold nutrients. These need to be added if this mix is all you use as your growing media, since while good coir has microbiology in it, it isn't soil and it doesn't have all the necessary nutrients.

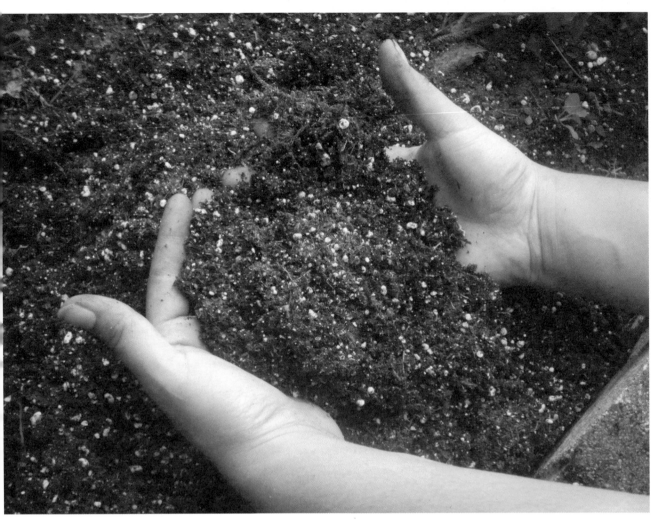

▲ Good soil for Autoflowering *Cannabis* should be light and fluffy. Addition of coir and perlite help. M. TULLOTTES, WIKICOMMONS.

Mixing soil with perlite and coir is, to many growers, the ideal. It does make a great growing mix, even if you might end up needing to also mix in nutrients. This depends on the soil you use, so evaluate the need after your first grow.

Biochar

One thing that helps ensure sufficient nutrients in a soil mix is fully

d and watch them grow!

teed Analysis

CONTAINS NON-PLANT FOOD INGREDIENTS

Active Ingredients: 1.35% – Mycorrhizae
(total of all species)

Endomycorrhizae – Propagules per gram

Glomus intraradices	0.6
Glomus mosseae	0.6
Glomus aggregatum	0.6
Glomus etunicatum	0.6

Purpose: The mycorrhizae may assist plants
with the uptake of nutrients and water.

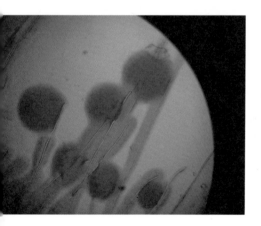

▲ *Rhizophagus intraradices*, the mycorrhizal fungus that forms a beneficial symbiotic relationship with Autoflowering *Cannabis*, is now available commercially. Note that a variety of older names are still in use because people once thought they were different fungi. The root here is the familiar tomato. JUDITH HOERSTING AND SAMSON90 (CCO), FROM WIKICOMMONS.

charged biochar because biochar is the perfect soil condominium for soil food web members. It consists of mostly carbon and has plenty of places to get away from the bigger predators.

Biochar has to be charged before using because the manufacturing process kills off life. Charging is accomplished by mixing it with, and storing it in, compost for a couple of weeks. Then add it to your soil mix.

MYCORRHIZAL FUNGI

There is really only one species of mycorrhizal fungus that forms mycorrhizae with Autoflowering *Cannabis*. As of this writing it is known as *Rhizophagus Intraradices*, but you may still find labels using *Glomus mossae*, *Glomus rhizophagus*, and *Rhizophagus irregularis*. This is the same mycorrhizal fungus that infects tomatoes, by the way, and can be used on those plants as well.

There are more and more brands of the appropriate mycorrhizal mix. You can find these in most nurseries and at all grow stores. The important thing is to check the expiration date to get the freshest.

GROWING CONTAINERS

Most gardeners find growing Autoflowering *Cannabis* is easiest when done in containers. They don't have to be fancy, just have drainage and be of adequate size for the life of the plant. This is because it can take a week for any plant to fully recover from transplanting. That is a long time for fast-growing Autoflowers.

The ideal size is between 10 to 20 liters (3 to 5 US gallons). Those ubiquitous hardware store buckets, with drainage holes added, are perfect. Woven cloth containers with handles are convenient, too. The exceptions to the 10 to 20 liters rule are the really diminutive varieties, which should be planted in 4 to 8 liter (1 or 2 US gallon) pots.

If you do plan on transplanting for some reason, then it is absolutely imperative you do so with the least amount of disturbance to the roots. The plant needs to reestablish its connection to the soil so it can mine for nutrients.

Remember (how could you forget!), Autoflowering *Cannabis* plants grow so fast that disturbing them really messes them up.

I repeat, for your first few grows, it is a much better idea to simply plant where your Autoflowering *Cannabis* will finish up life. Later, you can transplant to your heart's content, but in the beginning, make it a no fuss, no muss, and no disturbance grow.

The one caveat to the no-transplant rule is that you have to be careful not to overwater a large container before it is filled with roots. Too much water can drown a plant by making the soil anaerobic. Ensure very adequate drainage, which you should have anyway.

LIGHTS (AND MAYBE REFLECTORS)

Just because Autoflowing *Cannabis* doesn't respond to a photoperiod, doesn't mean you shouldn't grow it under the very best lighting conditions possible. Genetics, soil, and (finally) the third leg on the stool is proper light. Sure, you can grow at a windowsill, without extra light, but under lights your Autoflowering *Cannabis* plants will thrive. Use the best lights you can afford.

Depending on where you live, it may be easiest to grow outdoors at least for your first crop. Sunlight provides all the light your plants will need, and it is free, so it is perfect to see if you really want to get into this hobby.

Indoors, however, you really should provide your plants with the best supplemental light you can. Frankly, in large part thanks to growing larger *Cannabis*, there have been many advances in plant grow lights, and better and better systems are always being developed.

This is not a book on lighting. You already grow plants and understand the principles. I strongly suggest a trip to a grow store or even a lighting store. The options offered there will include all manner of fluorescent lights, LEDs, metal halides, plasma lights, and more. There will be the latest and greatest, sure, but also the cheapest and most efficient.

Seek sales advice and match up a system with what you can afford and need. Just realize that if you can grow tomatoes under a particular set of lights you already own, then you can grow Autoflowering *Cannabis* under them as well. Use these until you decide if you want to make an investment in something else.

I will keep it very simple. First, Autoflowering *Cannabis* plants go through two basic growing phases: vegetative and flowering. Blue light waves during the vegetative stage help keep plants short, with less distance between nodes. As a result, Autoflowering *Cannabis* plants grown with lots of blue light waves in the spectrum usually produce better.

Fluorescent lights like T5s contain lots of blue wavelength and can be placed close to plants. Metal halide lights are heavy in blue wavelength light, but they also produce lots of heat, so be very careful. They are also much more expensive. Wait until you see if you want to continue to grow Autoflowering *Cannabis*. (You will.)

Flowering requires red wavelength light. You can find bulbs for this too, but really, switching lights? That's too much work. In general, a full-spectrum bulb will work great for your beginning needs.

Incandescent bulbs—Incandescent light does not have the proper bandwidth for growing *Cannabis*. There is too much far red and infrared light, and growth concentrates in stems. The results are spindly and weak plants that don't really produce.

There are special incandescent bulbs that have had their spectrums tweaked to grow plants. However, these have to be kept close to the plants to provide enough light, and unfortunately, they are very hot and can easily burn the plants.

To be clear, I do not recommend that you use incandescent bulbs. They are not efficient. They are not effective.

Fluorescent tubes—Back in the day, you could tell someone was growing because fluorescent grow lights gave off a distinctive purple hue. It was the only fluorescent tube you could use for indoor grows until someone figured out you could take a 2-bulb shop fixture and outfit it with one blue and one red wave-emitting tube.

Today there are all manner of fluorescent lights under which you can grow Autoflowering *Cannabis*. Look for the old-fashioned tubes or the newer, thinner T5 bulbs. (T stands for tube and 5 for 5/8 of an inch diameter. The older styles were T8s and T12s, which were 1 and 1 ½ inches in diameter.)

Fluorescents are cheap, and they are easy to set up in a small space. There is little heat emitted so they won't burn plants. This is good because they need to be close to plants to be effective. Remember to make it easy on yourself and have an adjustable system that adapts as plants grow. With small Autoflowers, that does not take much.

A good combination for lighting, and probably the least expensive, is a cool white tube mixed with a regular warm tube. A cool white tube with a grow tube combination works well, too. There are lots of different spectrums offered in fluorescents. This is why I suggest you get help from a professional at a grow or a lighting store.

For starters, give fluorescents a go and see if you enjoy these plants. At the very least, fluorescents are great lights for starting seeds as they won't burn them.

CFLS—Do consider Compact Fluorescent Light Bulbs, CFLs. These fluorescents will screw into a regular incandescent bulb socket. They are very inexpensive and easy to find.

T5S—If you want a better light, but still want something that will enable you to grow in a small space, consider T5 fluorescents. These are finger-thick tubes that can be used horizontally over plants, as you would expect, but vertically as well. They are super-efficient and just right for growing Autoflowers.

LEDS—Arrays of light-emitting diodes, LEDs, are all the rage for growing these days. They are extremely efficient. For example, an LED bulb rated as 60W equivalent will actually use only about 12W.

They generate very little heat. They are easy to handle, being very lightweight. They also last practically forever.

Recently LEDs have become available with full-spectrum and other designer spectrum bulbs intended for use as grow lights. Some are available in the T5 format for use in T5 fixtures. Flexible LED tape is also available in grow light spectrums. These light tapes run off a 12V DC power supply and can be arranged imaginatively without fear of burns or electrocution. It would take a lot of light tape to provide stand-alone lighting for growing *Cannabis*, but at minimum such lighting could be used to supplement natural light. Ready-made LED arrays come in all sizes, perfect for single plants or, linked together, many.

HIDS—High Intensity Discharge Lights (HID) are what most commercial growers use. These are more like street lights than what a home gardener uses. They have great growing spectrums for *Cannabis* and put out massive amounts of light.

HID lamps are expensive. And, they generate a lot of heat which you will have to deal with. Both the lights and the fans will use lots of electricity. They can really grow great Autoflowering *Cannabis*, however.

Metal halide—Metal halide lights are also more like street lamps than they are like gardening grow lights. However, they can really pump out a high-quality light spectrum that can grow wonderful Autoflowering *Cannabis*. Metal halide performs best for plants in their vegetative state.

Metal halide lights are extremely inefficient, giving off a lot of heat—up to 15% of the power these lights use is given off as heat. The light they give off should be contained and reflected, or much of it will be wasted.

HPS—High Pressure Sodium gives off a yellow light that is terrific for flowering, but is hard on the eyes when used to grow plants. (These too make great street lamps.) They require relatively high voltage and thus need a ballast to adjust the current. They also contain a bit of mercury, which should give the grower some concern.

Like Metal Halides, HPS lamps give off light in all directions and have to be reflected. They will burn plants if they are anywhere close to the plants. They may require a growing room bigger than the home gardener wants.

Plasma—Plasma lights are the closest thing to actual sunlight. There have been tremendous advances in the technology behind these systems, and commercial growers are discovering the cost savings associated with their very efficient high-frequency, high-voltage power supplies and controllable, full-spectrum light. While there is not yet a small plasma system for home gardeners, at least one is in development. This is definitely a development worth tracking.

Reflect light for maximum efficiency

When it comes to Autoflowering *Cannabis*, it makes sense to get the maximum efficiency out of any supplemental lighting. Many lights come with reflectors attached, but lots don't. If yours doesn't, buy a reflector that will fit your particular situation. These really help get you the very best results, all other things being equal.

While not absolutely necessary, line your grow area with a reflective material. I don't advise you use store-bought aluminum foil unless you can keep it completely smooth, as crinkles can cause hotspots and actually burn your plants.

One great material is sold as reflective gardening film. It is white and reflects up to 70% of the light that hits it. You will also find mylar sheeting designed for lining grow areas. At the very least, consider painting the walls of your grow area white. This will reflect light.

TIMERS

Even though you won't have to worry about photoperiods when growing Autoflowers, you should use a timer if you are going to use lights. These plants can grow with 24 hours of constant light; however, in my opinion, they do best when given around 20 hours of light a day. Let the timer do the work of turning the lights on and off so you can get some sleep. After you get experience, you can come up with your own light schedule.

Timers are cheap. If you don't have one already, they are available from multiple sources including grow stores. They are easy to install and to use, and they make growing Autoflowering *Cannabis* plants easier.

NUTRIENTS

It may be necessary to fertilizer your Autoflowers. This depends on the condition of your soil and the genetics of your seed. Ideally, it contains all a grow needs and you don't need to fertilize.

If you do, there are all manner of organic fertilizers designed for growing Autoflowering *Cannabis*. Something like a balanced organic fertilizer such as 3-2-4 works great. This provides enough nitrogen for the vegetative stage and phosphorous during flowering. One feeding should be all that's required.

Since you really can't tell what is missing from a plant's diet, consider kelp for mixing in your soil, as it has all of the essential plant nutrients (and more) required to feed a soil food web community. Mix it in with your soils and compost, preferably a few weeks before you plant, and you may not need to provide any additional feed for your plants.

FANS AND ODOR CONTROL

You must supply ventilation to any indoor growing areas. You probably know from growing tomatoes that still air is an invitation to mildews and other pathogens. Circulating air is a great way to keep your plants healthier. It also aids in evaporation from stomata which encourages continual uptake of nutrients.

There many kinds of fans you can buy, but they basically break down into static and those that oscillate. Just make sure you pay attention to physics: provide both a source of air intake and some way for air to move out of the area.

You need to keep an eye on watering. The fan will cause the plant to take up moisture from the soil as water evaporates out of the stomata, drying out the soil more quickly.

The *Cannabis* industry has developed a number of ways to treat *Cannabis* odor should it bother you or anyone in the vicinity of your growing area. There are different sized charcoal filters that do a great job of removing orders.

You can get systems at grow stores that mix ventilation with odor control. Some growers use laundry softener sheets (though these are not organic). They put them at the air exit vents to sweeten the air. (Personally, I find this smell more offensive than the smell of *Cannabis*.)

PEST CONTROL

Hopefully, you won't have any pest problems. However, be prepared. Occasionally, Autoflowering *Cannabis* plants are attacked by pathogens, insects, mollusks, and other pests.

For fungal problems, neem oil is a great starting organic fungicide, as well as an insecticide and a miticide. In fact, since it is effective against such a wide range of problems, including powdery mildew, spider and broad mites, aphids, and white flies, neem (or one of the products that uses it) should be in your arsenal.

Neem is readily available in many forms and safe to use. The big drawback is its garlic smell, so you must be careful using it around buds and flowers. It is so very strong that it will negatively impact your plants' growth if you use it too often.

Horticultural oils can also be an effective and safe solution to control insect problems. They work by smothering the insect. They are only effective for a few hours so they should be applied often. As with neem oil, you don't want to get these on flowers. (I am betting they don't taste that good.)

Insecticidal soaps work in a manner similar to horticultural oils, though they are considered to be less hard on the plants. They are made from fatty acids, which weaken the shells of insects. You do not want to get them on flowers.

Spinosad products are made from an *actinomycete*, a soil microbe (specifically *Saccharopolyspora spinosa*). They are organic and safe, but usually only remain effective for 24 hours after mixing with water. They disrupt insect nervous systems, especially those of white flies and aphids.

Diatomaceous earth is comprised of microscopic fossils that have very sharp edges. Sprinkled on soil, it will rip and hold in place critters that come into contact with it. Use horticultural-grade product and don't breathe it in.

Predatory biologicals are available to take out a number of specific insects. You can find these at grow stores where you can seek advice as to which should be used. Or you can order them via the Internet. They are very effective, and some can carry on from crop to crop. Their disadvantage is that they limit other options, specifically sprays that might kill off problem insects.

HUMIDIFIERS

Ideally, you should maintain a humidity of around 55% (40 to 70% range) during the vegetative stage when growing *Cannabis*. Once the plants start to flower, however, it is best to drop it so that it stays below 50%. Once the buds open, lower it even more. It sounds like a lot of work.

High humidity, too much water vapor in the air, can actually stunt some plants' growth. Most importantly, high humidity is ideal for the growth of spores of the various fungi (molds) you don't want to infect your plants. *Cannabis* plants often first show signs of these molds in the developing flowers, which means that they don't become visible and a real problem until it is too late.

Optimal Humidity			
Clones 70-80%	Vegetative 40-70%	Flowering 40-50%	Final Weeks of Flowering < 40%

Too much moisture leads to mold, bud rot, & mildew! Make sure there's always a breeze moving over and under plants. If possible, keep humidity low as plants approach harvest.

◀ Humidity is important, but adding a humidifying system is usually not necessary. WINNI CASACOP.

I suggest you do not install a humidifier in your grow area unless you absolutely know you need to increase humidity with one. They are just too risky and usually cause too much moisture.

Instead, mist your plants frequently, which shouldn't be a problem because you should be observing them often. A simple household misting bottle will do the job.

In some situations, you might end up with too much moisture in the air. If your grow room is small enough or you are using a grow tent, use a bowl of rock salt to absorb the excess moisture.

TEMPERATURE

Autoflowering *Cannabis* development is delayed by cold temperatures. On the other hand, if it is too hot, plants shut down. As with tomatoes, it is difficult to get flowers to form and set at temperature extremes. For these reasons, an inexpensive thermometer will come in handy. Spend a bit more and get an inexpensive recording thermometer so that you can monitor the daily high and low temperatures.

Research suggests that the ideal temperature range for Autoflowering *Cannabis* is 24 to 30°C (75 to 86°F). Understand that growing indoors at the warmer end of that range has the impact of reducing humidity a bit. This is not necessarily a bad thing. What *is* a bad thing is to let the temperature get to 36°C (96°F). This will shut down the plant.

▶ Autoflowers are extremely sticky. Get small nail-trimming scissors from a drugstore and dedicate them for trimming. You may want to wear gloves. JUDITH HOERSTING AND CANNABIS TOURS, WIKICOMMONS.

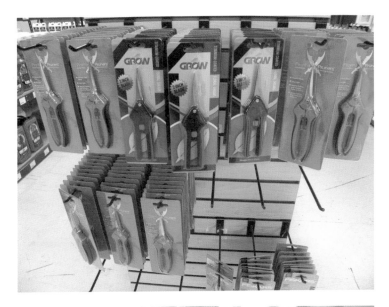

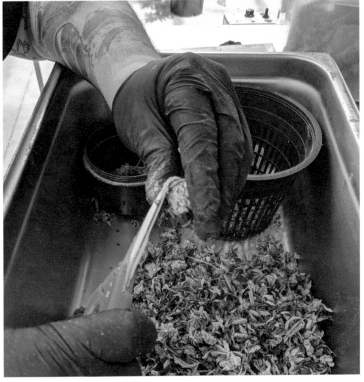

Remember, lights give off heat. And remember that this usually means a drop in temperature when they are off. Make sure the temperature doesn't drop more than 10 degrees, as this will create problems with your plant and stunt its growth.

You can find ways to adjust and maintain the temperature when growing indoors. Outdoors is another matter. Autoflowering *Cannabis* plants get used to temperature fluctuations that slow down indoor grown plants (which have acclimatized to ideal conditions) and can even survive a bit of frost (which may actually increase the production of THC). It is not worth taking any risks that could kill the plants, however, and absolutely isn't worth it during your first grows.

MAGNIFICATION VIEWING TOOLS

You will need some form of magnification to better observe the flowers of your crop and to help you determine the time of harvest. The go-to tool is a simple jeweler's loop. These cost under $10 US or Canadian. You can find them with magnification as high as 100x but much lower power, 5x or 10x, will do. Look for one that has a small LED light embedded into it, as this will come in very handy.

A second option is a USB microscope that you attach to a phone, tablet, or computer. These are a bit more expensive than the loops—you can find one for under $50 US. This may seem like overkill, but it will also give you the ability to take photos of insects and flowers.

If you have a cell phone (and who doesn't?), then you probably have a magnification app and that will work just fine. And, the macro lens in a digital camera is another great tool for magnifying your flowers to see if they are ready to harvest or to look for infestations of insects.

TRIMMING SCISSORS AND RUBBING ALCOHOL

Autoflowering *Cannabis* flowers are sticky. Very sticky. You will definitely need a dedicated pair of scissors to trim your flowers, so they can be dried and cured properly. The best are small scissors

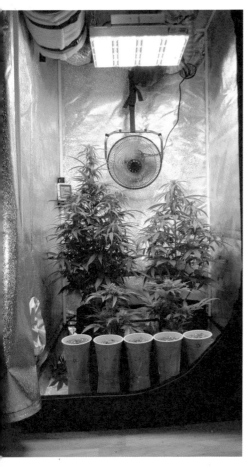

▲ Grow tents are not necessary, but they do make it easier to grow Autoflowering *Cannabis*, as they provide a self-contained growing area. You probably should wait to buy until you decide that the investment is worth it. FULL DUPLEX.

with very fine tips. They have to be small enough to snip off the tiny branches holding the flowers without damaging trichomes.

If you decide you like growing Autoflowering *Cannabis* plants, you may want to invest in an inexpensive hand bud trimmer. There are several on the market that do a fantastic job in much less time than it would take using scissors.

Rubbing alcohol is often used for cleaning trimming scissors. There are also special soaps designed to remove resin (great for cleaning your hands) as well as a number of contraptions designed to clean your scissors. (Necessity is the mother of all inventions, and for some reason, people in the *Cannabis* industry come up with interesting ideas!)

GROW TENTS

Grow tents are becoming all the rage for growing Autoflowering *Cannabis*. These reflector-lined tents can be used to grow a few plants, all neatly tucked away into one small area. If it were not for their price (from $75 to $250), I would include one in this list as a needed supply. Certainly, if you can afford one, a grow tent can really help you and your plants achieve maximum efficiency.

Some grow tents come fitted with LED lights and pots, and all you have to do is add the plants. Most can accommodate 4 Autoflowering plants. You can make your own. Just remember that you will need vents to let the air in and out.

OTHER SUPPLIES

Glass jars for curing and storage are a must. As noted, there are terpenes that dissolve plastic, but do not react to glass. Tightly sealing lids are a must to keep air and humidity out, both of which degrade cannabis.

Yellow sticky traps make a great deal of sense if you have flying insects. Make sure you hang them just above the plants so they will be effective.

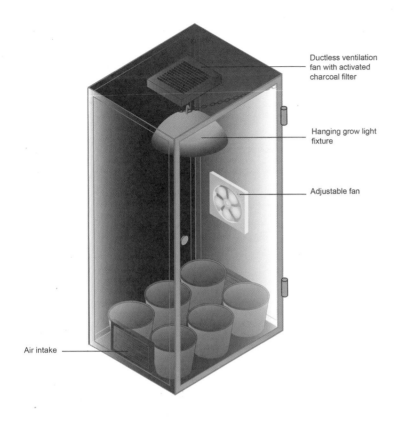

Ductless ventilation fan with activated charcoal filter

Hanging grow light fixture

Adjustable fan

Air intake

◀ A simple grow tent diagram.

WINNI CASACOP.

Simple Light Box

In sum, this book is predicated on how easy it is to grow Auto-flowers as a hobby plant. Add things to the list that will make it more enjoyable for you.

KEEP IT SIMPLE

Once you have located both seeds and supplies and made a decision as to where you want your first grow, it is time to see if growing Autoflowering *Cannabis* is really as much fun and as rewarding as growing tomatoes. You don't need to buy lots of stuff. Just treat your plants like the tomatoes you grow every spring.

4

LET'S GROW SOME AUTOFLOWERING *CANNABIS*

YOU HAVE ENOUGH information. It is time start growing your first Autoflowering *Cannabis* plants.

There is a reason that the slang name for *Cannabis* is weed. You can simply plant a seed, walk away, and it will probably grow into a plant. It is that easy. If you want a better plant, however, you need to pay just a bit of attention.

Follow my directions until you can take full measure of this plant. Learn the ways of Autoflowering *Cannabis* just as you did the tomato, and growing them will become second nature (and just as easy). Later, you can experiment with different growing procedures to match your own particular experience, needs, and conditions. Remember to check your regional laws and rules on how many plants you are allowed to grow.

Finally, I am going to assume you are growing in a container and indoors for the purposes of this chapter. Obviously, growing Autoflowering *Cannabis* directly in the garden is not that different. Nor is growing outdoors on a deck. It is the same plant. The big advantage is that you do not need lights outdoors. The disadvantage is that you cannot control the temperature and humidity.

Growing Autoflowering *Cannabis* a whole process, not just one point in time such as, say, when you harvest flowers (or try them).

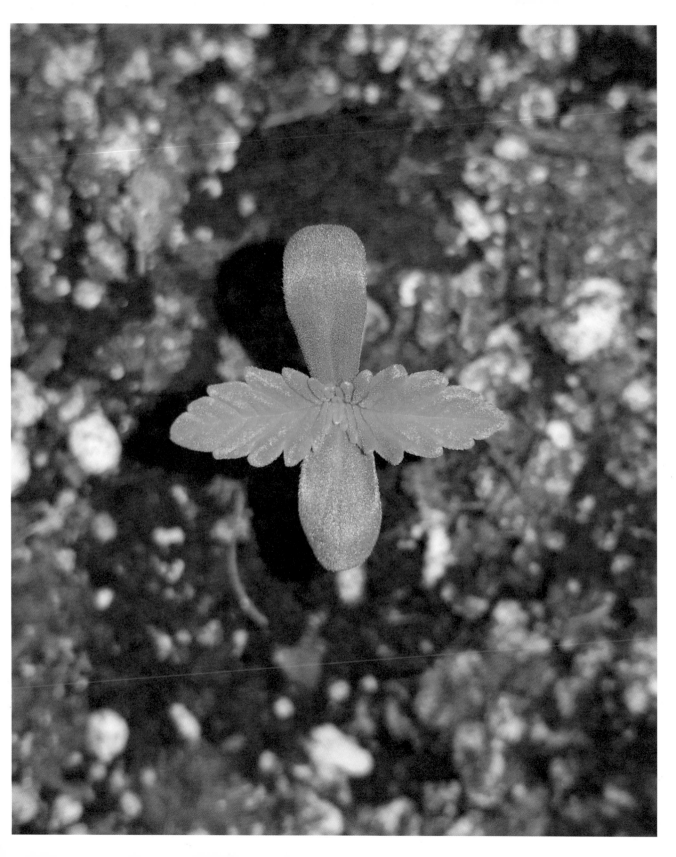

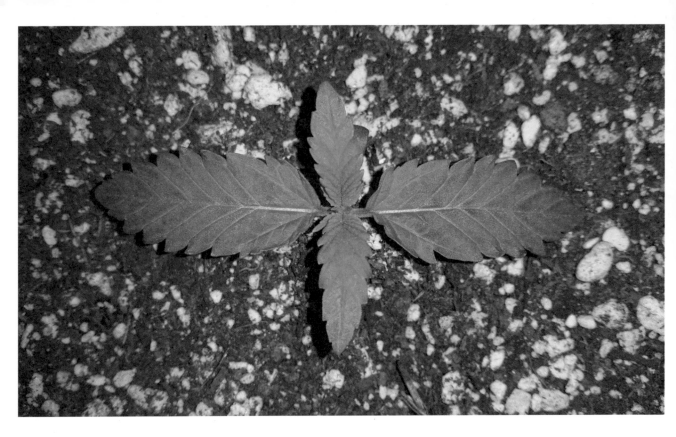

▲ Ripley's Day 7. GBD/DAZ MEPHISTO.

These are amazing plants. Their rapid growth, alone, makes them unusual and fun. Growing them should be a journey (and an engaging one at that).

LIFE CYCLE OF AUTOFLOWERING *CANNABIS*

Here is a quick overview of what to expect over the course of the plant's life. This is followed by a more detailed discussion of the steps necessary to get there.

From germination to 2 weeks

Germination of seed planted directly in soil can take up to 5 days, but usually happens rapidly, between 24 to 48 hours after the seed is exposed to water. The seedling opens as the plant's taproot sprouts

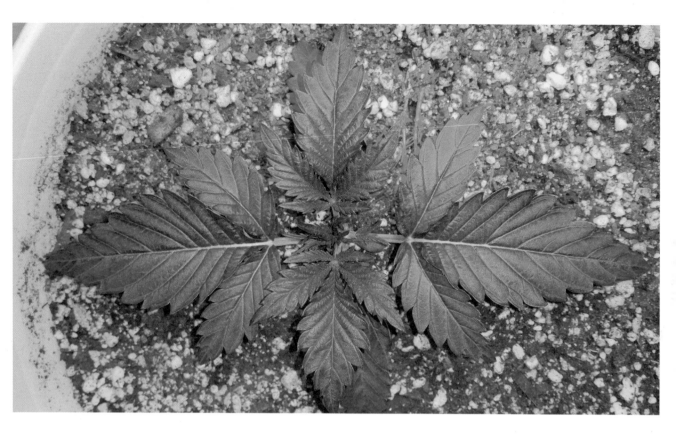

▲ Day 12. GBD/DAZ MEPHISTO.

and elongates. The two cotyledons, so-called seed leaves, are followed by the first set of true leaves. The second set of leaves quickly follow and then a third, all within an extremely short period of 10 days or so.

Each successive set of briskly growing leaves has more of the characteristic serrated fingers, with the third set finally looking distinctly *Cannabis*-like. It is at this stage that the desired hormones are fully active in the growing tip. If plants are going to be trained, this is when to start.

Below ground, the root system is developing and spreading into the soil mix. The plant's exudates are attracting and supporting a working soil food web. Signals are also being sent to *Rhizophagus intraradices,* the mycorrhizal fungi you added to the soil mix, inviting them to invade root hairs and enter a symbiotic relationship.

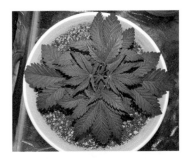

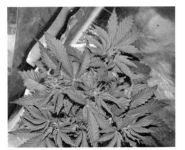

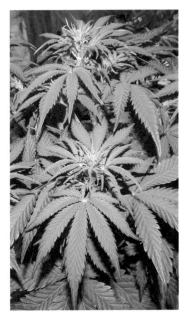

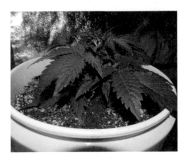

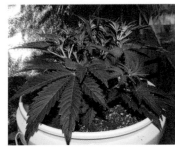

▲ Day 18. GBD/DAZ MEPHISTO. ▲ Day 23. GBD/DAZ MEPHISTO. ▲ Day 28. GBD/DAZ MEPHISTO.

From 2 to 6 weeks

The plant quickly puts on vertical growth with increasing internodal distances. Depending on variety, a growth rate of 4 cm (1.5 in.) a day can be achieved. You can see the plants growing. At the end of this phase, the plant is up to 1 meter (3 ft.) tall if it is of the super Autoflowering types, or at full height of around 18 inches if it is a regular Autoflower.

White pistils appear as early as the third week and continue to show up through week 5 depending on variety. Flower buds develop. The plant is putting everything into growth, and it is hard for it to keep up, so it may look a bit dull. Keep an eye on it for any drastic color or leaf changes—otherwise, a loss of some green color is normal.

From 6 to 8 weeks or so

Growth slows and blooms (female, though possibly male) grow bigger. Side buds appear and grow. The plant's aroma strengthens as

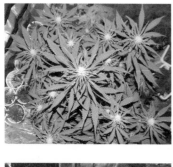

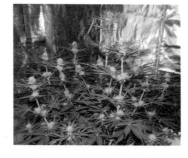

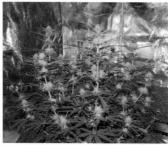

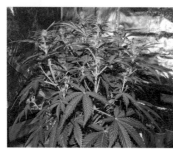

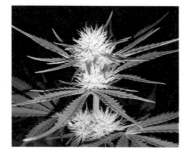

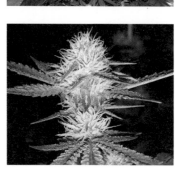

▲ Day 33. GBD/DAZ MEPHISTO.　　　▲ Day 39. GBD/DAZ MEPHISTO.　　　▲ Day 44. GBD/DAZ MEPHISTO.

trichomes develop. At the end of the period, some clear trichomes start to cloud up. Individual pistils start to turn brown.

Growth slows and the plant may green up a bit as it is finally able to keep up with nutrient demands. If the plant continues to lose its green color, add nutrients—just once and diluted, of course.

From 8 weeks until harvest

Trichomes start to turn from clear to cloudy to amber. The vast majority of pistils turn from white to brown. The top flowers usually ripen about a week ahead of lower flowers that continue to develop.

The big early fan leaves lose color because there are not enough nutrients left in the soil. These leaves should be removed. Harvest is near.

All the pistils turn brown, and the trichomes become milky. It is time to harvest. Some gardeners will want to wait until 20% of the trichomes are amber. Others, until more are amber, depending on the desired cannabinoid to THC ratio.

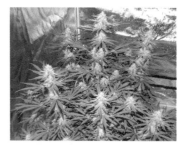

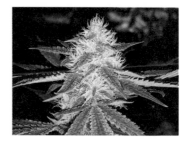

▲ Day 50. GBD/DAZ MEPHISTO.

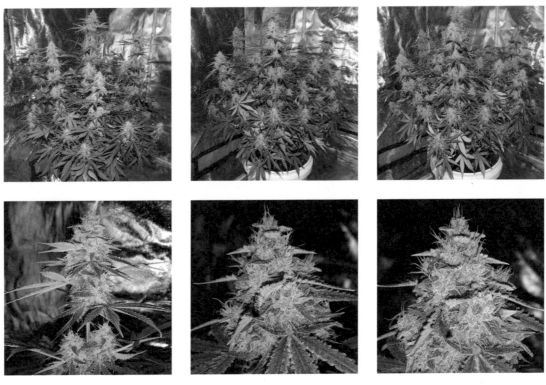

▲ Day 55. GBD/DAZ MEPHISTO.   ▲ Day 60. GBD/DAZ MEPHISTO.   ▲ Day 65. GBD/DAZ MEPHISTO.

TEMPERATURE

Autoflowering *Cannabis* seed germinates best at 25°C (77°F). Consider using a heat mat (just like you would when starting your tomatoes). Room temperature is fine, although it may take a bit longer for the seedlings to emerge.

Once germinated, Autoflowering *Cannabis* does best when grown in a temperature range between 24 to 30°C (75 to 86°F). Again, these are perfect temperatures for tomatoes. Night temperatures really shouldn't drop below 10°C (50°F) even though the plants can survive at cooler temperatures.

Keep water temperatures in the same range as the ambient air temperatures (which is easy: set aside a bucket filled with water). This way you won't shock roots or the soil food web that surrounds them.

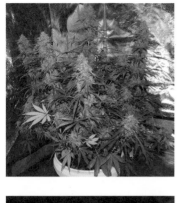

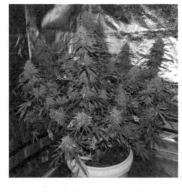

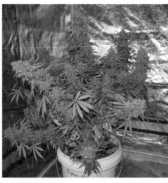

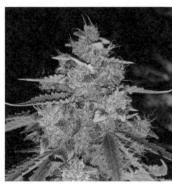

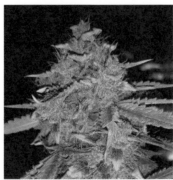

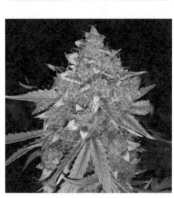

▲ Day 70. GBD/DAZ MEPHISTO.

▲ Day 75. GBD/DAZ MEPHISTO.

▲ Day 80. Harvest Day!
GBD/DAZ MEPHISTO.

GERMINATE SEEDS

There are a number of ways to germinate an Autoflowering *Cannabis* seed. All it takes is for the seed to be able to absorb water through its shell. Any way you can germinate a tomato seed will work for starting Autoflowering *Cannabis*.

The easiest method to germinate an Autoflowering *Cannabis* seed is to poke a hole in damp soil about 25 to 38 mm (½ to 1½ in.) deep. Use your finger or a pencil. (Isn't this how most of us start tomatoes and other vegetables?) Cover the seed with soil mix, and a seedling should emerge within 2 to 5 days.

A variation of this method is to use a seed starting wafer, the kind used for tomatoes and other vegetables. Comprised of compressed soil, coir, or various mixes, they expand when wet. Stick a

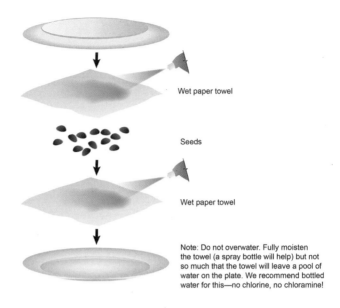

Wet paper towel

Seeds

Wet paper towel

Note: Do not overwater. Fully moisten the towel (a spray bottle will help) but not so much that the towel will leave a pool of water on the plate. We recommend bottled water for this—no chlorine, no chloramine!

▲ Plate/Paper towel germination method. WINNIE CASACOP.

seed in and wait for germination. They usually hold enough moisture so you don't need to add any water for several days.

Of course, these methods can be a hit-or-miss proposition, as with any vegetable seed started this way. But Autoflowering *Cannabis* seed is relatively expensive. To insure more certainty in germination, two other methods are suggested.

The first is to drop a few seeds into a glass of warm water. After 12 hours, start checking the seeds. As they absorb water, they will split open, revealing a tiny bit of white taproot. By the end of 24 hours, you should notice this happening to all your viable seeds. It is time to plant (but only after "rolling" or otherwise applying mycorrhizal fungi to the root).

A second method begins by putting the soaked seed on a damp, unbleached paper towel. (Some skip the 24-hour soak in a glass of water, but don't for your first couple of attempts.) Cover these seeds with a second damp towel or fold over the first towel to cover them.

Cover the seeds and toweling with a second plate. Alternatively, put the damp towel into a plastic baggie and store this in a dark, warm location.

Once seeds are in the damp towel, wait another 24 hours before carefully checking on them. You can leave seedlings in this setup for up to 5 days, but it is best to plant as soon as there is a discernible root, so root hairs develop in the soil and do not grow into the fibers of the towel.

The argument for soaking is that it lessens the seeds' exposure to air during germination and this prevents "damping off," a fungal attack that will kill the seedlings. Unless you live in a humid climate or have had problems germinating seed before, I would not be overly concerned, but providing air ventilation and air movement are good preventative measures.

APPLICATION OF MYCORRHIZAL FUNGI BEFORE PLANTING

Always use mycorrhizal fungi, *Rhizophagus intraradices*, to inoculate the seedling. If you are germinating seed directly in the soil, then roll the seed in the fungal mix first. This will coat the seed with enough propagules of the fungi. The fungi will establish itself in the root and soon start to mine the soil for nutrients to feed the plant.

Autoflowering *Cannabis* plants grow so fast that applying mycorrhizal fungi may not be as effective as it is with the slower-growing *sativa* and *indica*. Nonetheless, the inexpensive cost of the fungi (versus the potential returns) makes its use very worthwhile. And, if you are using a cover crop of sorts, the fungi should help it grow and perform as well.

PLANTING

Your soil should be watered and drained before you plant so that you don't have to add (much) water right after you plant. Adding water post planting might wash away seed, will change seed depth in the soil, and might wash away some of the mycorrhizal fungi propagules.

Just to insure mycorrhizae, make sure you mix the fungal preparation into your soil. This way, new roots will grow into it and be inoculated.

If, after you have grown a plant or two, you feel the need to add organic fertilizers to your soil, then before planting is the best time to do it. If you are using a good soil mix, then your plants won't need additional nutrients until later in their life cycle, so add nutrients out of the initial root zone: fill the pot ⅓ full, lay down nutrients, and then add the rest of the soil. This will allow the plant's roots to grow into the nutrients by the time the plant needs them.

When planting a germinated seedling, don't touch the rootlet, as this may damage the delicate root hairs. Hold the seed by the shell or the cotyledons if they have appeared. Very carefully place the seed (or seedling) in the hole, 25 to 38 mm (1 to 1½ in.) deep. Sprinkle enough soil to fill up the hole.

If the seedling has a long root tip, make an impression with your index finger so you can place the root on its side (but at the right depth). After topping off the planting hole with soil, spray just a bit of water on the hole to gently (and naturally) tamp down the soil, ensuring contact with the seed and the emerging root.

WATERING

The most difficult aspect of caring for any plant, be it tomato or Autoflowering *Cannabis*, is watering. Check your plants every day. Keep the water pH at 6.5 and at room temperature.

Too much water and your plants will literally drown at the roots, and the soil food web will be starved of necessary oxygen as well. Too little and your plants won't be able to feed themselves and maintain cellular turgor (hydrostatic pressure). In addition, the soil food web goes dormant. The rule that guides your watering is to just pay attention.

How much water do you need to give your plant? During active growth, Autoflowering *Cannabis* can use a lot of water. A good rule of thumb to start with is to use enough water to equal 20% of the size of the container in which your plants are growing. By way of example, if you use a 5 US gallon container (19 liters), the 20% rule would mean that you apply 1 gallon (3.8 liters).

As to *when* to water, there is no hard-and-fast rule. Do what you do with tomatoes: stick your finger into the soil. You are looking for moist as in a cake, not wet as in a pie.

All in all, the Goldilocks rule applies: you don't want the soil too wet or too dry. Still, if you want a formula to keep you on the straight and narrow, weigh your pot daily. When its weight drops 20%, water again. Do the finger test before and after, so you will learn to feel when the plant needs water.

While on the subject of watering, most books suggest you keep the humidity at 80% during the seedling stage, about the first 10 to 15 days. This can be accomplished with a humidifier system, but it is better to make a temporary greenhouse over your seedlings with plastic, jars, or whatever it takes. Then, once the plants get into the vegetative growth stage, removing it will lower the humidity. Ideally it should then be between 55 and 70%.

FEEDING

The point of using good soil is to eliminate the need to constantly feed your plants. After a couple of grows, you will have a feel for how they grow and are supposed to look, and if your soil mix is doing the job.

What a blessing for the gardener that Autoflowering *Cannabis* plants grown in good soil simply don't need much by way of supplemental nutrients. In fact, use 1/8 to 1/4 strength fertilizer if you have to feed your plants. Too much nitrogen can cause leaf growth at the expense of flower development, which is obviously not great for yields.

Of course, there are limits to how much nutrient matter soil can supply. The first limit is how much of the necessary essential nutrients the soil actually contains. Hence the need for a test. Information is power. I advise you get one, especially if you are using your own blend.

The second limitation is the volume of soil. A large container has more soil for roots and fungi to mine (but can be more difficult to water properly). This is another reason to get good information from the seed supplier, so you will know what size container to use.

The third limitation is the pH in the vicinity of the roots. All gardeners know maintaining the proper pH is critical because if it is not in range, nutrients are locked up, unavailable to your plants. Again, a test is critical. It is the only way to know your soil's pH.

If your soils test well for nutrients and pH or if you buy a reliable commercial soil mix, you might be able to grow your first Autoflowering *Cannabis* without ever adding fertilizer. For the first grows, keep a close eye on your plants. There will be a slight dulling of the green seedling as it dashes into growth, but this is normal. A dilute ⅛ strength solution of a balanced organic fertilizer may be in order every other watering.

Feeding Tips

For the first two weeks, Autoflowering *Cannabis* plants are incredibly sensitive to feeding. Doing so can actually put the plant into shock. And you do not want to do anything to slow down the establishment of mycorrhizae, which overfeeding can do.

Autoflowering *Cannabis* plants grow so fast that they initially use lots of nitrogen, and lesser amounts of phosphorus and potassium. Some organic sources of N include seabird and bat guano, as well as blood, fish, and poultry meals. There are lots of liquid organic blends available.

Once the plant starts flowering heavily, phosphorus is the primary element most needed. Phosphorus deficiency results in leaves darkening in color, turning a brownish or purplish blue. You probably do not have to add phosphorus to your soil when growing Autoflowering *Cannabis* (the *Rhizophagus intraradices* specializes in seeking and obtaining phosphorus for your plants), but if you do, use good organic sources only. These include fish bonemeal, and colloidal phosphate.

Note that too much nitrogen during the flowering phase will result in lower THC content. By the same token, if you give your

Autoflowering *Cannabis* plants too much phosphorus during the growing stage, the mycorrhizal partnership stops. Delivery of Fe, Cu, K, Zn, and Mn can be impacted.

Potassium deficiency is indicated by an overproduction of side branches, which could be great, but they will be spindly and weak. This is in part because the plant will have trouble taking up Ca, Fe, Mg, Mn, and Zn. Potassium controls the stomata, so a lack of it can cause them to stop working and results in leaf curl. Potassium can be supplied with an application of potash, actually wood ashes. Seaweed and manures also contain K.

Again, you may not ever need to fertilize your plants, but you should know when a plant is in need and what to do about it. The solution is to hit the soil with diluted (⅛ strength) liquid organic fertilizer. Your plants need to respond in a day or two at the most, so solid foods don't help. A 3-2-4 ratio is suggested by commercial New Breed Seed and is a great starting point for home growers.

LIGHT

Autoflowering *Cannabis* plants do not need specific photoperiods. Lighting is still extremely important. There are two aspects to consider. The first are the number of hours of light. These plants can obtain CO_2 during the day, so they really do not need any darkness. You can grow yours under 24 hours of light. Many insist this is how to get the most from Autoflowering *Cannabis* and takes advantage of their special ability to flower regardless of the hours of light or dark versus their cousins which flower only after nights start getting longer than days.

Having grown some of these plants at 15 hours of light, I can tell you that is not enough. In fact, around 18 seems like a minimum, and more surely does not hurt. The theory of 24 hours makes sense, but something in me suggests giving the plant a few hours of rest. Experiment, but for your first grows, go with 20 to 24 hours.

Outdoors, grow your plants in full sun. Just remember that if started indoors, you have to harden off your plants to survive the wind and UV rays of the outdoors to prevent sun and wind damage. Keep your plants in the shade for a few days and then gradually move them into full sun over the next week.

Next, consider the intensity and coverage of light. Keep plants as close to the light source as possible without burning them. Expose the entire plant (or collection of them) so as to give maximum exposure to all the growing tips. This is where reflectors come in handy as does a reflective coating to walls, floors, and ceilings.

TRAINING

Commercial growers have discovered that training the branches of *Cannabis* to form more colas can greatly increase yields. This is done by pinching back the plant to create more active nodes or by exposing lower nodes to more light.

You may want to train your Autoflowering *Cannabis* plants, though I don't suggest it for the first grows. The breeder of your seeds has most probably worked hard to develop a plant that does not need pinching or training to produce enough flowers for an acceptable harvest. Only once you know what to expect (that is, what the plant looks like, how it performs, and the yield produced), should you consider pinching and training Autoflowering *Cannabis*.

Should you decide to experiment later, there are a few methods of training. Each has its advantages and disadvantages, and it is fun to experiment with them, but again, none of these may be needed.

One thing to keep in mind is that it is a good practice to tuck the large upper fan leaves under side stems. This will expose the lower nodes to better light with noticeable results. It is not really training, as you have to keep doing it.

Topping, High-Stress Training

The first and most popular way to train to increase yield is pinching off the plant's growing tip. This cuts off the supply of auxins (from the apical stem tip) to the lower nodes, allowing the plant's lateral buds to break dormancy and grow. (To belabor a point, the same thing happens to tomato seedlings.) Each pair of node tips, located on opposite sides of nodes below the pinch, responds. Each tip develops a new stem which will produce its own cola.

Pinching is easy: once a plant has developed 4 nodes (or 5 or 6), simply take off the growing tip. Amazingly, this will cause the seedling to develop 8 (or 10 or 12) new tips. They all grow and develop flowers as each strives to produce seeds.

Usually varieties that have grow time to recover, i.e., the ones that require more days to mature, do best with pinching. Again, look for information in the cultural directions provided with the seed.

Low-Stress Training

There is a second method to try and increase yields that doesn't slow the plant's growth nearly as much, if at all. This is low-stress training, LST. There are several different methods.

One method is to simply tuck the big fan leaves underneath and behind branches and stems. This exposes the flower tips to light. It can be done gently so that the leaves still can serve their function.

Another method is called FIM (for Shucks, I Missed). Instead of taking the whole tip off, only the tip's leaves are pinched or cut off (which must be why it is comparatively low stress). This causes four colas to form in replacement. If done to shoots at the 3rd or 4th node, you get a very bushy plant. FIMing on Autoflowers, while setting them back during recovery, is not as hard on the plant as is topping. Still, it is not suggested for first grows, even though you might want to experiment later.

In a much less energy-draining procedure, a plant can be simply bent and twisted, with nothing snipped or cut off (although often plants are pinched first and then trained using a low-stress method). This is like pulling a tomato down. Tomato plants and *Cannabis* will respond to this treatment in the same way.

Bending a stem confuses the plant as to where the top should be, and it sends auxins to nodes along the stem in an attempt to keep the plant in flowers, as long as the stems don't start to grow upward

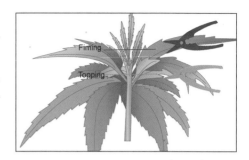

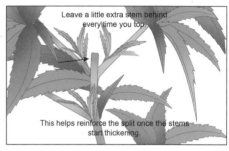

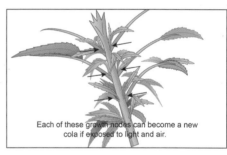

▲ Pinching or high-stress training.
WINNI CASACOP.

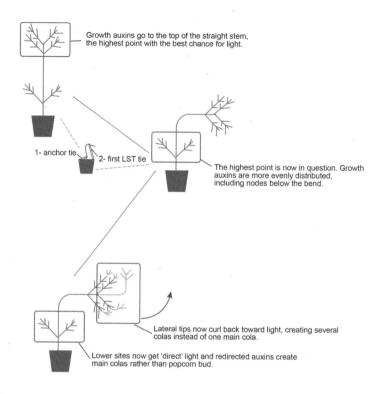

▶ LST Bending method.

WINNI CASACOP.

Growth auxins go to the top of the straight stem, the highest point with the best chance for light.

1- anchor tie 2- first LST tie

The highest point is now in question. Growth auxins are more evenly distributed, including nodes below the bend.

Lateral tips now curl back toward light, creating several colas instead of one main cola.

Lower sites now get 'direct' light and redirected auxins create main colas rather than popcorn bud.

Low Stress Training

again. In the case of Autoflowering *Cannabis* plants, the idea is to gently pull the plant stems into a more *horizontal* position so that all its nodes are directly exposed to the same amount of light.

LST methods—There are a couple of established procedures that use low-stress training. The first is known as SCROG or Screen of Green. This consists of placing a net over the plant so it grows into it.

Once a stem starts to grow through the netting, it is pushed back down under the net, bending it horizontally. This causes the auxin movement previously discussed, and new growth from these nodes grows upward through the net.

Another popular method of low-stress training is to train branches using string, yarn, bonsai training wire, or hemp twine (if

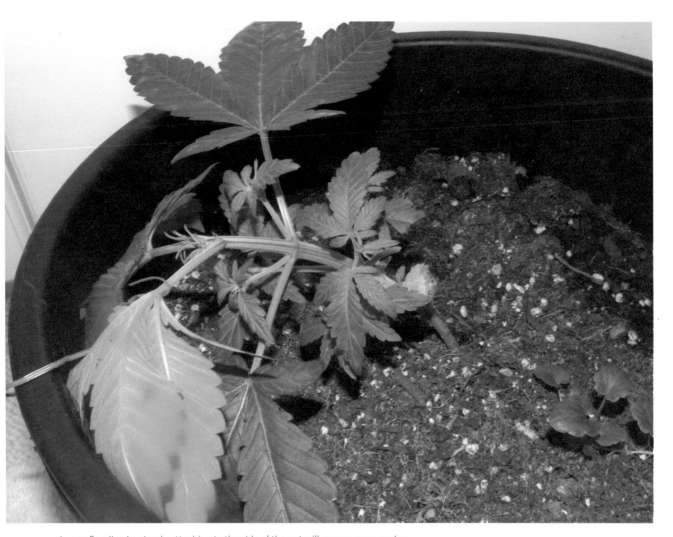

▲ LST Bending by simply attaching to the side of the pot will expose more nodes.

you don't think the plants will be offended). Tie the string to the first branch, gently bend it to the side of the container, and secure it there with tape or a binder clip.

Some growers use pots with holes drilled into the lip and secure the string through these. You should continue to train new branches all the way up to the first week or so of flowering, when the plant will stop elongating.

Circular LST ties the branches down in a circular or spiraling fashion. Not all Autoflowering *Cannabis* can handle this. It is an

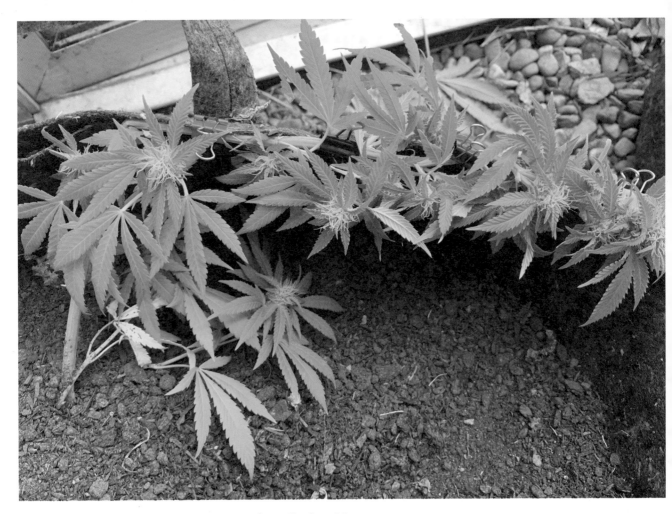

▲ LST Circular training. JUDITH HOERSTING.

easy way to maximize exposure to light and to increase yield to a maximum but may require the removal of a few leaves. It is pretty easy if you know the trick: the plant should be started at the side of the container so it is easier to guide the branches along its edge.

After the tip starts growing vertically again (a day or so later), make a second tie down and so on, eventually pulling the branch around the pot. You can clip the branch to the side of the container to help train it. You will end up with a beautiful arrangement and should have great yields, all other things like genetics and lighting conditions being equal.

This is possible because when Autoflowering *Cannabis* is young, the branches and stems are easy to bend without damaging them. If they do snap, just leave them as they probably will slowly repair themselves.

However, as the plant matures, stems become stiffer and you have to be more deliberate and slower in training. Then it may take a couple of days to pull a branch all the way down. And, because these plants go to flower so quickly, there is a point after which it doesn't make sense to train any further. Experience will guide you if you decide to engage in training at all.

The advantage to this LST method is that it is simple. It does not require any special equipment. You can also get creative as you learn the way these plants grow.

If you want to train an Autoflowering *Cannabis* plant, start soon after the emergence of the first set of true leaves. Over time, after you have grown a few crops, you will intuitively know when you can perform LST and what to expect from it.

Again, you may never need to train an Autoflowering *Cannabis* plant. The plant's breeder may have taken care of it for you.

JUST PAY ATTENTION

Keep an eye on your plants, checking them daily, at least. Keep some notes so you don't forget. Watch the addition of leaves, the appearance of sex parts, branching, changes in color, speed of growth, and all the other things discussed here.

Look for the pests and plagues that can hit any plant. Don't let plants dry out. And, if you see a need, then fertilize.

WHEN AUTOFLOWERING
CANNABIS IS READY TO HARVEST

Harvest timing can impact the characteristics of your flowers. Fortunately, there are clear signals given off by Autoflowering *Cannabis* to indicate the proper time. First, as the wanted compounds accumulate, the liquid in a plant's trichomes turns milky or cloudy. Then, all

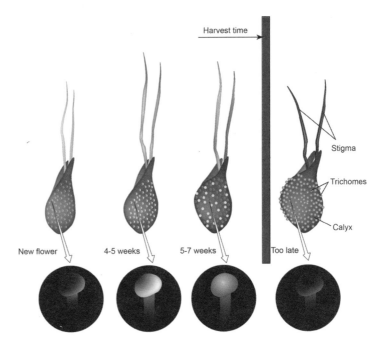

▲ Using stigma and trichomes to determine harvest time. WINNIE CASACOP.

the trichomes gradually turn a darker color, best described as honey or amber.

Harvest with early trichome clouding, and the high should be more energetic. Most commercial growers believe that at 70% milky trichomes the high is at its greatest intensity, with the highest amounts of THC. Lots of CBD is produced by the time 60 to 70% of the trichomes are amber, and the high is said to be less energetic and more sedative.

At the same time, as the trichomes color up, the white stigma curl a bit and start to turn brown. These alone are not a reliable indication of time to harvest, however. They can turn brown when touched during the growing process (so don't touch them, no matter how tempted), and water and cold temperatures can also prematurely brown them. Nonetheless, they can help indicate harvest timing, so you need to watch them.

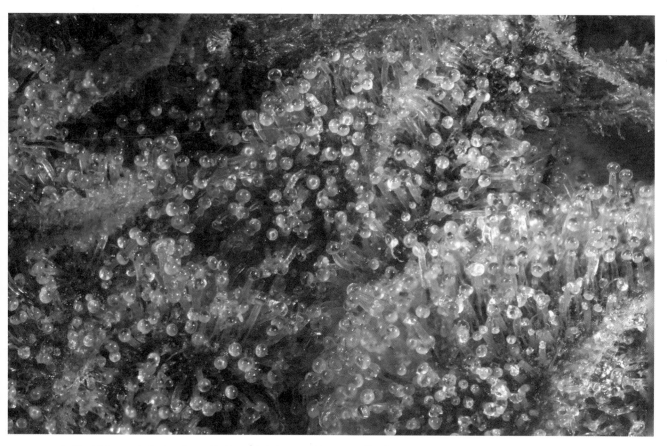

▲ The trichomes indicate a flower that is ready to harvest. Most are milky. Some are amber. FRED GUNNERSON, SOFRESHFARMS.

All things considered, once 50 to 90% of the stigma are brown, it is time to check out the trichomes with the hand lens. For your first grow, start checking trichomes when 25% of the stigma are brown. Remember not to touch the buds while doing so, if at all possible, as those trichomes are fragile.

It is best to use a magnifying glass or a small hand lens, your cell phone, or the closeup setting or macro lens on a digital camera to gauge trichome and pistil color changes. Finally, there are several inexpensive microscope attachments for your computer that will show your flowers on a screen. Do use some sort of magnification when determining harvestability.

Note that if (God forbid!) a plant continues to mature beyond the point of harvest, trichomes will turn gray and start to fall off. This would be 2 or 3 weeks after the first trichomes cloud up. It is doubtful you will ever let it happen—in any case, you shouldn't.

Autoflowering *Cannabis* flowers often do not all ripen at the same time. The flowers closest to the light are ready first, which makes sense. This means you must look at several flowers through magnification when making a harvest decision. It also means you should only harvest the buds that are actually ripe.

Finally, ripeness is in the eye of the user. As you become experienced, you will find that somewhere on the spectrum of trichome and pistil color will be your perfect harvest. Just remember, too early or too late and you are not going to get the maximum benefits of these plants, insofar as cannabinoids and terpenes are concerned.

A FEW FINAL WORDS ON GROWING

That's it. Autoflowers are truly easy plants to grow. Nature and breeders have ensured nothing about it need be complicated or difficult. Now, just grow some. That is the best way to learn how. Go ahead, without fear. Don't bother to train or pinch the plants. Just provide light, water, and the proper temperature and humidity.

Be ready to add additional nutrients if the plant calls for it. Keep notes. These days, that includes taking lots of pictures with your cell phone or digital camera.

You've probably grown tomatoes without much instruction. Let that give you the comfort you need to get growing Autoflowering *Cannabis*. If you have a problem, treat it just like you would, well, a tomato.

Once you see a female flower or a pollen sac, you won't forget the way they look, and it will become easier to recognize them in future grows. And once you see how these plants operate, you will automatically (just like recognizing the appearance of their flowers) know what to do. It *is* just like growing tomatoes, as I keep saying.

Finally, don't skimp on drying and curing. This is what makes mere ditch weed turn into fine *Cannabis*. It pays to set up a system and follow it. It takes a bit of patience, and you must not rush things. Oh, and, most important, have fun.

5

PESTS AND
OTHER POTENTIAL
PROBLEMS

AUTOFLOWERING CANNABIS is a plant, and there is always an insect or disease trying to take any plant out. (They want to live, too.) Be prepared, is the motto, especially when growing a fast-moving plant like Autoflowering *Cannabis*.

Actually, one of its saving graces *is* that Autoflower plants grow very fast. Pests can miss their opportunity. And, Autoflowers don't require specific hours of light to bloom. This means that if you have problems you cannot fix, you can always start over and almost catch up, rather than having to wait for a few seasons to roll around so you have the right photoperiod.

PESTS THAT LIKE AUTOFLOWERING *CANNABIS*

All plants can get attacked by pests, and Autoflowering *Cannabis* plants are no exception. Fortunately, the inclusion of the scrappy *Cannabis ruderalis* in their genes gives Autoflowering *Cannabis* plants some resistance. And, breeders are always working to improve upon their plants' natural abilities to grow pest-free. These efforts, and fast growth, make it difficult for some enemies to take hold or have an impact when they do.

There are lots and lots of books on plant pests, and as a gardener, you should have at least one as a reference. Still, there are some specific rules you should follow to prevent or minimize pests

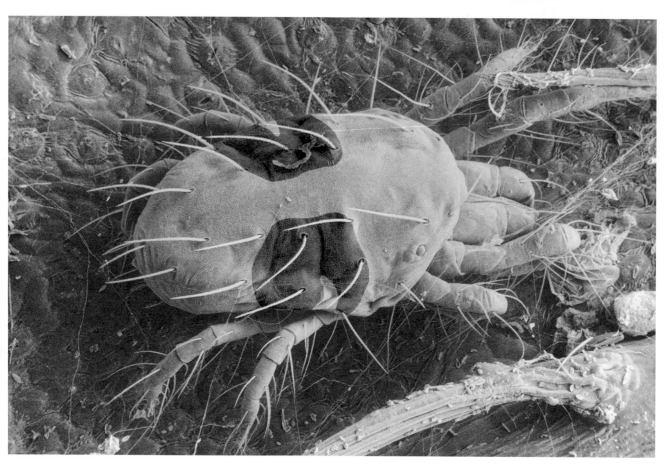

▲ The two-spotted spider mite, *Tetranychus urticae*, is one of the most common mite species of agricultural importance. If you see fine spider webs on your house plants, you probably have spider mites. USDA, ELECTRON AND CONFOCAL MICROSCOPY UNIT.

on Autoflowering *Cannabis*, and there are some specific critters that merit special note.

As a gardener, you already know that prevention is the best route. Keep your grow and grow areas clean, provide adequate air movement, and watch the humidity. Prevent pests.

Some specific pests

Here are the major specific pests for which you should be on the lookout. You are probably familiar with most of these as most can attack tomatoes (and other vegetables). Knowing what they look like is important. So is knowing what the proper organic remedy is to prevent or control them.

Spider mites—The two-spotted spider mite has a particular fondness for any *Cannabis*. These tiny (0.5 mm, 1/50th of an inch long) cell-sucking insects can be the bane of growing Autoflowering *Cannabis*. Here is where your hand lens will come in handy.

First signs of an infestation of mites are tiny white or orange spots appearing all over leaves, which then turn yellow. If you turn these leaves over, you will see tiny eggs and the characteristic webbing created by spider mites. It is most pronounced at nodes. The buds of badly infected plants will also become covered with the webbing.

Since spider mites thrive under hot and dry conditions, temperatures should be kept below 27°C (80°F), and the humidity should be controlled. Many commercial growers apply a mist every few hours. You might use a spray bottle a few times a day.

Help prevent spider mite infestations by keeping your growing area clean. Don't bring in other plants. If outdoors, don't kill beneficials by spraying any generalized insecticides. Keep plants in a constant breeze as this makes it more difficult for the mites to reproduce.

To kill spider mites, use commercially available neem-based products or Spinosad. Read the instructions carefully so you know how long the formula lasts and when to reapply. Mites are tough little critters. They are so tough that you really should toss your soil after the current grow and thoroughly clean everything.

Biological control employs the predator *Mesosaeiulus longipes*. This is an aggressive mite that works quickly. *Phytoseiulus persimilis* works well and is also available commercially. Lady bugs and another spider mite destroyer, *Stethorus punctillum*, are also available to reduce mite populations, though these probably only work indoors. If you use biologicals, you need to be careful as they can impact other wanted predators.

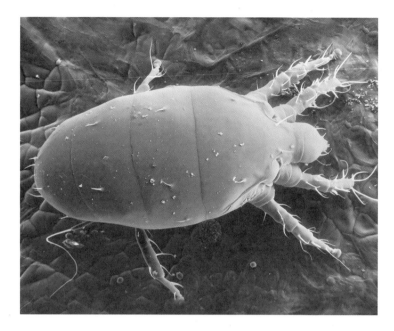

Grow stores will have lots of products from which to choose. Spray the entire grow area, the plants, soil, and containers. An effective home remedy spray for spider mites is a mixture of 9 parts water and 1 part rubbing alcohol.

Russet and broad mites—These tiny (0.5mm, 1/50th of an inch long) insects also suck the juices from leaves and stems. They are almost impossible to see, even with a good hand lens or microscope. Look, however, for first signs of wet or glossy-looking leaves that curl or develop drooping leaf tips. Later the leaves turn yellow and bronze and drop off. If plants are in flower, (alas) these will turn brown and die.

Russet and broad mites are very hard to eradicate as they lay their eggs *inside* the plant. Neem oil is the first recommendation. The predatory mites *Neoseiulus Californians* work well and are less harsh on the plants. A fungal remedy is MET52, *Metarhizium anisopliae Strain F52*, available from grow stores. Aloe products won't kill them, but mites will avoid aloe and move to treated trap plants such as broad beans.

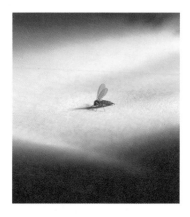

Heat may help you deal with russet and broad mites. If you can safely heat your grow area to 46–49°C (115–120°F) for an hour, you can do wonders. So will 10 seconds of water at 60°C (140°F) degrees. It is difficult for any mite to survive that. Obviously, you will need to remove your plants first as it is difficult for them to survive the heat, too.

Fungus gnats—These tiny flies breed in the top layer of soil. They mine roots which stunts plant growth, and they are very annoying as they fly around. Fungus gnats are attracted to and thrive in soil that has been overwatered and are normally not a problem if you let the soil surface dry out in between watering.

Aiming a fan on your soil will speed up drying and make it harder for gnats to move around. A physical barrier made by covering the soil with newspaper or a cut paper bag prevents adults from getting into the soil and laying eggs.

Organic solutions again include neem oil. Products containing *Bacillus thuringiensis* var. *israelenisis* (Bt) work great as well. They are best when applied while watering. *Stratiolaelaps scimitus* lives in the soil and will take out larva. You can also spread diatomaceous earth on the soil.

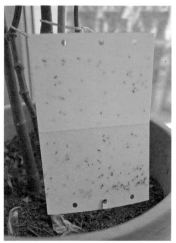

▲ Fungus gnats. JEZEBELITHACA AND BY ICH, WIKIMEDIA COMMONS.

White flies—Tiny white flies lay eggs on the undersides of leaves. After they hatch, the larva suck the juices. Their numbers can become quite large. Often you won't notice them until the population increases and all of a sudden you see lots of adults flying around. In addition to these annoying swarms, you will note leaves yellowing and a general decline in the health of the infested plant.

Treat white flies with neem oil or Spinosad products. You have to repeat applications as white flies are difficult to fully eradicate. When you spray, cover soil and the growing container. If you are growing indoors, parasitic *Trichogramma* wasps can be used to control populations.

Powdery mildew—White spots and powder on leaves are the signs of powdery mildew, a fungus that attacks Autoflowering *Cannabis* and eats leaves. A few fuzzy spots soon spread to other leaves. Infected buds are unusable. If you grow tomatoes, you have probably seen it. It can coat a plant in a matter of days.

Spores of powdery mildew are in the air, but they are encouraged by high humidity as moisture is needed for the fungus to grow. Good air circulation makes it difficult for the fungi to get established so using a fan is a good preventative measure.

If your plants are hit by powdery mildew, reducing humidity to below 45% is a must. It is also imperative that you have a change of air, not just movement. Isolate your plants so they don't spread the disease.

Early detection is key. Once you find it, immediately use a spray made of any of several home remedies: Baking soda (30mL/3.8 liters or 2 tablespoons/gallon of water), milk (1 to 9 parts water), hydrogen peroxide (mix 5mL of 35% strength hydrogen peroxide to 3.8 liters of water, or 1 teaspoon/gallon). Neem oils as per instructions are some of the best commercial remedies.

Aerated compost tea sprayed on leaves is a good prophylactic move. The microbes in the tea take up space and nutrients that would have been used by pests.

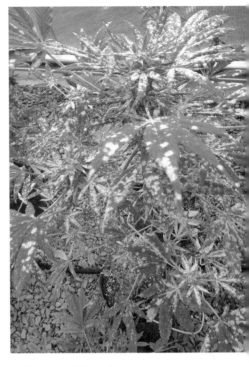

▲ Powdery mildew on leaves. HAROLD FRAZIER, NEW BREED SEED.

Botrytis is another fungus that attacks Autoflowering *Cannabis*. It causes damping off of seedlings, weakens and destroy stems, and, most heart breaking, can infect and kill flowers. (Ah, the injustice of all that waiting, only to have them cut down in their prime!) It is hard to spot until established with a gray, white, or blue-greenish mold growing on the inside of the flower bud.

Look for signs of *Botrytis* in flowers. It starts with a drying leaf sticking out from a cola. And keep looking even when the flower has been harvested and is drying. This is a real pest, and if you get it, you will need to clean up to get rid of the spores. The best bet is to prevent it by making sure you have good air circulation.

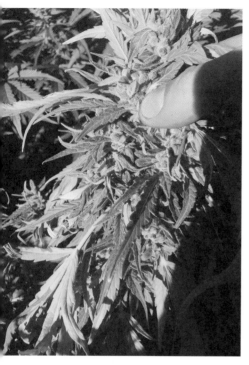

▲ *Botrytis* takes out a large cola.
HAROLD FRAZIER, NEW BREED SEED.

Slugs and snails—Slugs and snails decimate leaves, starting with characteristic holes. They weaken plants and can destroy flowers. Besides, they leave a slime trail. These are particularly nettlesome when growing Autoflowering *Cannabis* outdoors.

The use of black felt cloth containers helps keep them from getting to plants. Trapping works great. Put beer or yeast water in shallow containers to attract them away from plants. Place these next to containers or just outside your gardens, not in them. Diatomaceous earth makes a great barrier as neither of these pesky mollusks likes to move over sharp edges.

Other pests—Other pests that may impact your plants include scale, caterpillars, crickets, grasshoppers, leafhoppers, leaf miners, mealybugs, thrips, and nematodes, to list a few familiars. There is plenty of information about all of these on the Internet or at your library.

The most important takeaway is to keep your eyes open for pests. Observe and inspect your plants often. Act quickly and follow instructions.

GENERAL RULES TO DEAL WITH PESTS

Autoflowering *Cannabis* plants are no different than other annuals, and the same rules apply when it comes to pests. Inspect your plants every day. It isn't that difficult. You should be making observations and gathering information about your plant's growth all the time anyway. Taking pictures with a cell phone is a good practice. That way you can go back, if you do have an infestation, and find and learn to recognize the very early signs.

Second, pests spread, and they spread quickly. Immediately remove any plants that are infected and either destroy them or keep them isolated while you treat them. Some problems will be serious enough or far enough along that you really do need to cut your losses, so to speak. Don't unnecessarily put your other plants at risk.

And third, always stay organic, starting with biological solutions when applicable. One of these is squishing large insects by hand. You can also try to remove insects with air (either blasting them or using a small hand vacuum cleaner) or use a water spray to knock them down. Resort to chemicals, and just organic ones at that, only when you absolutely have to. Again, make sure to follow directions precisely.

It should go without saying that a gardener should never spray Autoflowering *Cannabis* flowers with even organic pesticides unless growing for seed. Some go one step further and never spray any part of the plant when a plant is in flower. To do so risks having spray drift onto flowers, and that can impact the quality of the harvest.

If directions allow, always repeat applications, even though you cannot see any more pests. Pests hide. And, vary the remedies as well, if possible. Autoflowering plant pests quickly develop resistance if you constantly apply the same remedy.

SOME ORGANIC SOLUTIONS TO DEAL WITH PESTS

One of my favorite tricks to deal with insect pests, specifically spider mites, whiteflies, and thrips, is using broad beans as trap plants. A couple of plants grown in a separate pot and placed among Autoflowering *Cannabis* plants will act like a magnet to attract pests away from your crop.

Broad beans, *Vicia faba,* will at least serve as monitors of any potential problems and, because of the short life of Autoflowering *Cannabis,* may actually keep things in check. (Plus, you may even get some green beans.) One side benefit is that broad beans are legumes, and the plants will put nitrogen into the soil.

Finally, a certain number of pests is okay. This is because of the speed at which Autoflowering *Cannabis* develops. The pests just don't have enough time to multiply to sufficient numbers to destroy your crop. Still, you will not want to carry over these pests to future grows. Cleaning up after each harvest is extremely important to meet this goal.

NUTRIENT DEFICIENCIES

Autoflowering *Cannabis* plants grown in good soil may not need supplemental nutrients. There is nothing unusual here; your plants

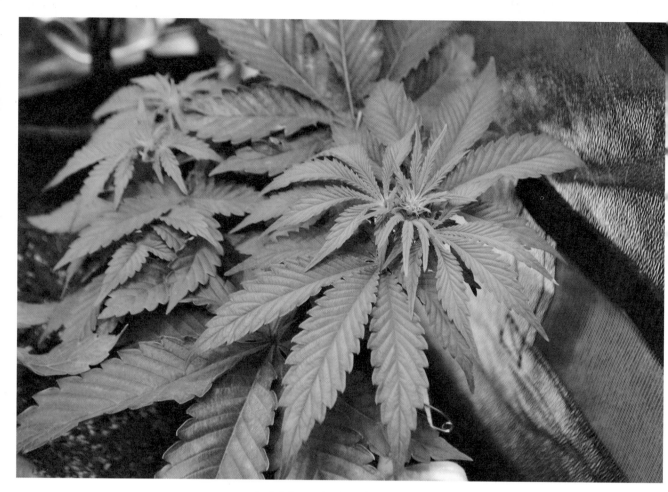

▲ Autoflower showing calcium deficiency (at top of photo). FULL DUPLEX.

will only falter if there is something missing in the soil mix. This is why I stress buying soil from a local grow store to start, based upon the recommendation given there.

Gardeners don't like to hear that you cannot really tell what nutrient may be lacking just by looking at leaves. A lack of any one of three major nutrients can cause yellowing of leaves, for example.

Still, leaf signs tell you something is going on. Just exactly what is an educated guess. Leaf changes are where to start looking. (If you want more information about this subject see *Teaming with Nutrients*, Timber Press, 2013.)

Boron deficiency—Boron is needed for cell wall development and for development of flowers, among other things. The tips of plants that are experiencing boron deficiency exhibit yellowing of leaves. They then turn brown and eventually gray. This is the key tip (pardon the pun). Since very little boron is needed by plants, a deficiency is a rare occurrence.

Calcium deficiency—Calcium is needed for building cell walls and it helps plants absorb potassium. There are two key plant signals for this deficiency. A lack of calcium results in weak branches that fall off. Leaves display dead patches that get larger as time passes.

Chlorine deficiency—Chlorine is needed for the proper operation of stomata and is needed to break the bonds of water during photosynthesis. It is rarely in short supply because it is in our water; but, when it is, leaves turn bronze.

Copper deficiency—Copper is used in the production of sugars and proteins. Signs of a deficiency are seen in new leaves, which will display dead leaf tips and leaf margins. The leaves will take on a darker blueish color. They curl and die.

Iron deficiency—Iron is needed to pass around electrons during key metabolic processes needed for nitrogen fixation, and is also used in making chlorophyll. Plants that are lacking in iron display yellow leaves, starting with new growth and upper leaves. The leaf veins will remain green. Leaves start to fall off.

Magnesium deficiency—Magnesium is in the center of the chlorophyll molecule, so it is absolutely critical for photosynthesis. When lacking, the plant's lowest leaves turn yellow and die. The signs move up the plant as younger leaves also begin to die.

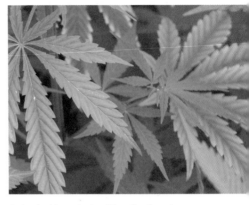

▲ Lack of iron starts with yellowing of new growth. So does a lack of nitrogen and zinc, but this plant probably has iron deficiency. DIYANA DIMITROVA OF DEPOSIT PHOTOS.

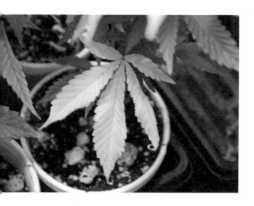

▲ Autoflowering *Cannabis* showing signs of nitrogen deficiency. Note the green veined leaves on the left. This is the early sign and distinguishes this yellowing from that caused by other problems. CANNABIS UNIVERSITY.

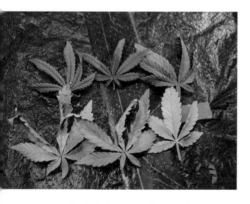

▲ Autoflowering *Cannabis* leaves showing progression of phosphorus deficiency. FULL DUPLEX.

▶ A simplified nutrient deficiency chart. WINNI CASACOP.

Manganese deficiency—This is a key nutrient, as it frees oxygen during photosynthesis. If it is in short supply, new leaves develop dead spots and then turn yellow.

Molybdenum deficiency—This nutrient is needed for plants to use nitrogen properly. Leaves in the middle of the plant turn yellow. New growth curls and twists, and sometimes the leaves turn a maroon or crimson color.

Nitrogen deficiency—Nitrogen is used for the production of proteins and enzymes, among other things. If a plant is deficient, it will turn yellow. This usually starts with the older leaves which give up nitrogen for new growth.

Phosphorus deficiency—This is the key element in ATP, the energy currency of plant cells. The symptoms of phosphorus deficiency start with the darkening of foliage. Growth slows and leaves turn purple and brown and curl upward.

Potassium deficiency—Potassium is used to control stomata, in photosynthesis, and for water transport throughout the plant. Deficiency results in lower leaves turning brown and dying. This is often preceded by faster growth, which is pretty hard to notice in Autoflowering *Cannabis*. Stems can take on a reddish color.

Silicon deficiency—This element is used to protect plants from insects, among other things, so symptoms of deficiency can include more attacks than usual. In addition, since it helps with photosynthesis, plants that lack it become weak and spindly.

Sulphur deficiency—Sulphur is needed for the production of chlorophyll. If a plant lacks adequate supplies, new growth turns yellow. Growth slows and becomes stunted.

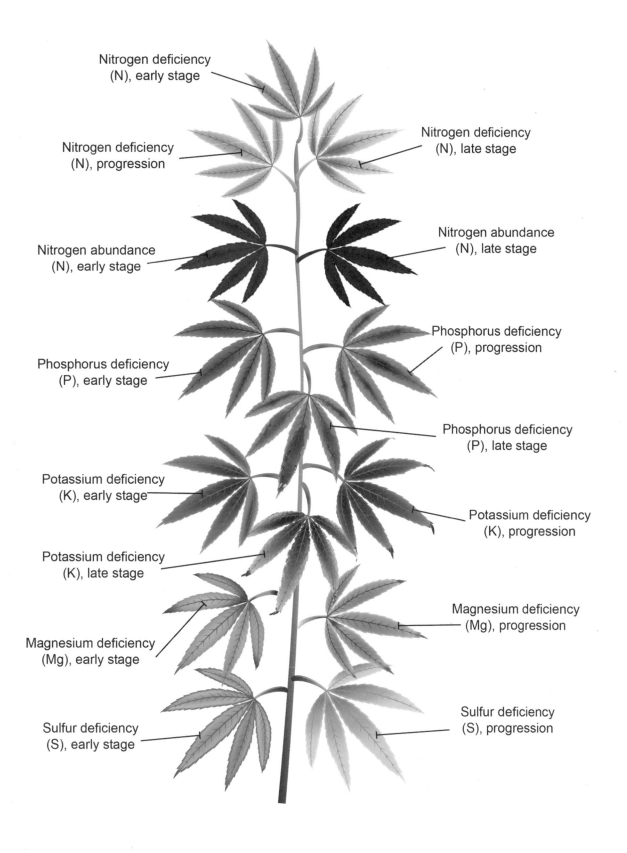

Nitrogen deficiency (N), early stage

Nitrogen deficiency (N), late stage

Nitrogen deficiency (N), progression

Nitrogen abundance (N), early stage

Nitrogen abundance (N), late stage

Phosphorus deficiency (P), progression

Phosphorus deficiency (P), early stage

Phosphorus deficiency (P), late stage

Potassium deficiency (K), early stage

Potassium deficiency (K), progression

Potassium deficiency (K), late stage

Magnesium deficiency (Mg), progression

Magnesium deficiency (Mg), early stage

Sulfur deficiency (S), early stage

Sulfur deficiency (S), progression

Zinc deficiency—Zinc is a key component of many enzymes and in the production of auxin, a key growth hormone. Without enough zinc, plants leaves become twisted. Veins on older leaves turn yellow.

DEALING WITH NUTRIENT DEFICIENCIES

Yellow leaves with or without dark veins, wilting, leaf curl, dark and dead spots... all of these can be caused by nutrient deficiencies. Autoflowering *Cannabis* plants show many of the same symptoms as do tomatoes. You can find them depicted by searching the Internet.

As with pests, preventing nutrient deficiencies is much better than having to correct the nutrient balance in your soil, especially while trying to grow a plant in it. Corrections take time, depending on the nutrient, and you may not have enough time to be effective with these fast-growing plants. For this reason, it is important to use the absolute best soil you can find. Either it should be already tested, or you should test it yourself to make sure it is not deficient in any of the essential nutrients.

A great thing about growing Autoflowering *Cannabis* is that it doesn't take much soil mix. This means you can afford to buy the best, or you can make your own best mix. It also means you should toss it into your compost pile or into your gardens when you finish a crop, as you can afford to start over with new, fresh, fully nutrient-filled soil.

Remember that soil pH is important when it comes to nutrient availability. Ideally it should be between 5.5 and 6.5. If you buy your soil, chances are this is the range it is in. In particular, if the pH is too high, iron, zinc, copper, boron, and manganese become locked up. If the pH is too low, it is phosphorus, calcium, and magnesium that are unavailable. Testing soil pH is easy and inexpensive.

Finally, the use of cover crops can help keep the soil food web functioning and add nutrients, especially nitrogen, to your soils. Some will also fight off or trap pests. My favorite is white sweet clover. Most other common cover crops are too big for Autoflowering

Cannabis. It is best to start these plants early so they are established when you plant your Autoflowering seedlings.

ABIOTIC PROBLEMS

In addition to pests and nutrient deficiencies, there are a few other common problems you should be aware of when growing Autoflowering *Cannabis.* These are the same problems you encounter growing tomatoes and vegetables, so they shouldn't come as a surprise to the experienced gardener. Still, it doesn't hurt to give you a reminder.

Overwatering and underwatering

This is particularly a problem with seedlings. Too much water literally suffocates the roots. Too little and the plant cannot take up nutrients and may not be able to maintain turgor (or stiffness), causing it to wilt before it dies. Keep the soil surface slightly moist until the second or third set of leaves appears. Then let the plant tell you what it needs.

Humidity and temperature

Autoflowering *Cannabis* is negatively impacted by both too high and too low humidity and temperature. Plants become stressed and stop growing. THC production is lowered.

The ideal temperature for growing Autoflowers is 26°C (78°F). You can vary this a bit, but once you hit 32°C (90°F) and above, plants slow and stop growing. At the other end of the spectrum, Autoflowering *Cannabis* can survive at temperatures around 7°C (45°F), but they may change color at lower temperatures, taking on a dark reddish hue. They also won't grow very well.

Low light quality

Autoflowering *Cannabis* seedlings will stretch and elongate unnaturally when the light is not strong enough. This is a natural response for any plant, but these grow so fast, it is accentuated. When branches develop, they are hard to support on skinny stems. It is important to give your plants as high a quality of light as you can.

Seeds won't germinate or are not feminized

Sometimes Autoflowering *Cannabis* seeds won't germinate. And when they do, sometimes, when they are sold as feminized, they produce male plants instead of just females. These seeds are expensive. If either of these problems happens, try to retrieve your money from the vendor who sold them. For failed germination, also try soaking them in a 4-to-1 water to regular 3% hydrogen peroxide mix. Some believe this will break the seed hull, while others contend it works because it kills harmful bacteria that prevent germination.

When males appear from a packet of feminized seed, there isn't anything you can do to change things. Let the supplier know and consider trying to breed your own plants using the male pollen. There is no guarantee the progeny will carry the autoflowering gene, but it might be fun to try your hand at breeding since you have some male pollen.

Soil drains poorly

No plant likes its roots to sit in water. If your soil won't drain, your plant will slow and eventually die. Increase air circulation. By the same token, soil can drain too fast and plants won't get nutrients. Consider carefully removing the plant without disturbing its roots and placing it into better soil.

NOTHING NEW

If you are an experienced gardener, there is really nothing new to learn when it comes to pests and protecting your plants. For the most part, you will already know what to do. And, with any luck, you won't be tested.

Finally, if something goes wrong with your plant, it is not worth risking your health trying to fix things. This is a plant that you probably plan to ingest. There is no place for dangerous chemicals. If you can't fix things safely using organics, then toss the plant. It goes without saying that this is a hobby. Keep it a safe one.

6

HARVESTING, DRYING, CURING, AND STORING

I KEEP SAYING THAT it is easy to grow Autoflowering *Cannabis* plants. By your first harvest, you will know it really is true.

Unfortunately, you can't simply pick flowers off an Autoflowering *Cannabis* plant and use them. There is a use for green tomatoes, and you can eat ripe ones right off the vine. Not so, *Cannabis*. The crop has to be dried.

Do not ruin your crop at this point. When and how you harvest those flowers will have much to do with the quality of your grow. So will drying and manicuring and curing. These are the finishing touches, and they greatly influence how your harvest will look, but even more important, how it tastes.

Do not rush things at this stage. If you do, you will not be able to achieve the quality of product you want. This is one way in which Autoflowering *Cannabis* differs from tomatoes.

HARVESTING AUTOFLOWERING *CANNABIS* PLANTS

Harvesting is simple. The flowers on the tops of Autoflowering *Cannabis* plants usually ripen first. The lower part of the plant and smaller limbs will have flowers that may take a week more to ripen. This is why you may not want to simply rip the plant up and start the drying process as you would with the larger *Cannabis* relatives.

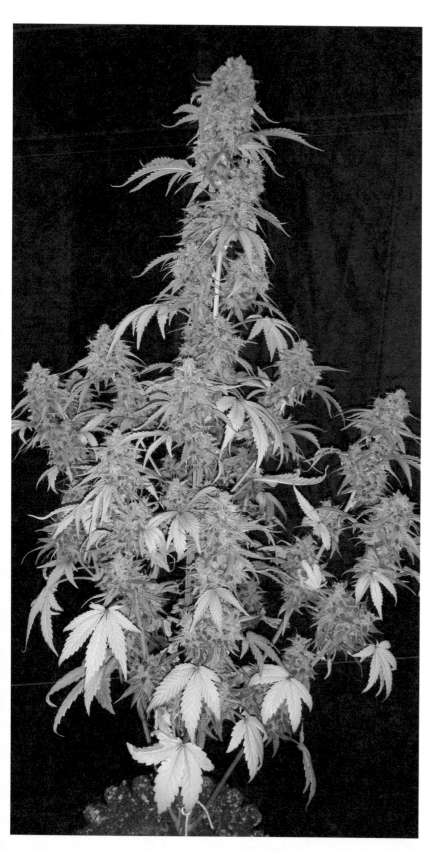

◄ Ripley's OG, Ready to harvest, Day 70. GBD/DAZ MEPHISTO.

Depending on genetics, however, and how the plant is exposed to light, it is possible for all flowers to be ready. When this happens, cut down the entire plant and dry it before trimming off the flowers.

For the first grows, harvest when trichomes are half cloudy with some amber for energetic highs, 70% milky trichomes and more amber ones for the greatest intensity of THC and energetic highs, or for more sedative highs, wait until 70 % of the trichomes are amber.

Make sure to include as much stem as possible when you harvest stems as this will make it easier to hang them. Often it is easier to remove the top colas all at once. This has the benefit of exposing unripe flowers on lower side branches. Then just keep an eye on these remaining flowers and remove them when they reach the stage you have chosen.

In any case, before you cut flowers off a plant, carefully remove the larger fan leaves. Toss these into the compost unless you are going to make oils or bubble hash, both of which are beyond the purview of this book but instructions for which can be found via the Internet.

Actually, you shouldn't touch the flowers at all. This is a rule. Remember, those glandular trichomes are fragile. Do not cause them to degrade any more than they do naturally.

DRYING THE HARVEST

Drying Autoflowering *Cannabis* is necessary as it removes the plant's grassy chlorophyll taste. Your crop needs to be evenly exposed to air so it will dry. Drying also removes water from the flowers' cells. These are the same reasons tobacco is dried.

Drying will prevent mold from destroying your crop, but the crop remains susceptible to mold while it is still damp. It is a good idea to check a drying harvest every few days to make sure things are progressing without molding up. If any mold is found, remove infected buds and increase air circulation.

The goal to drying is to remove 75%, or so of the water from the flowers. How to tell if you have accomplished this? You could weigh a representative cola or flower (or even the whole crop if you can do it carefully without damaging the trichomes) on a postal scale. Then calculate 75% of that number. Keep re-weighing the cola until its weight is reduced 75%. This gets a precise reading, but the handling can damage trichomes.

Fortunately, there is a much easier method. Just bend a drying branch or twig. If it snaps, the harvest is ready. If it doesn't snap, it is not ready. Again, be very careful not to handle flowers lest you damage trichomes.

There is such a thing as drying too quickly. In that case, the taste will remain grassy. Be patient. It takes at least a week to get the chlorophyll to break down enough to make a difference. Depending on conditions, drying can take about 5 to 15 days.

Do not be tempted to use heat to speed up drying. Microwaves and heat both degrade THC. In fact, these are not even worth trying, no matter how convenient and tempting it may be.

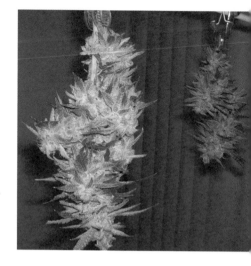

▲ Hanging some nice bud to dry using a hanger and inexpensive clips. PSYCHONAUT, WIKICOMMONS.

Hanging

The easiest way to dry Autoflowering *Cannabis* is to hang your harvest in a dark spot where there is air circulation. The temperature should be between 15 and 27°C (60–80°F). The humidity ideally should be 50%. There should be no direct light, and actually, darkness is much preferred. Easy.

You can hang your harvest in a cardboard box, open drawer, a closet, or the like. Clipping to coat hangers works great, too, as the whole crop can be easily moved.

The hanging process is where drying can be speeded up. Ensure good air circulation to remove the moisture that evaporates and to prevent molds attacking the still damp plants.

The brown paper bag trick

A drying method used in humid areas is so easy and so effective that it is my go-to method for beginners and advanced Autoflowering *Cannabis* growers, no matter what the humidity. Any brown paper bag will do the job, provided it isn't coated with wax.

Place your harvest on the bottom of the bag so that no individual piece touches another. Flowers touching each other increase the chances of fungi (aka mold) growing. Mold is the enemy of your harvest. Don't fill the bag, only lay down a single layer.

Carefully close the bag by rolling down the top a couple of inches. Use a binder clip to keep it shut. There should be plenty of air in the bag. The brown paper will absorb the moisture from the flowers.

You can place bags on several layers of newspaper (if you can find any!) to absorb this moisture or, better, hang the bag. Either way, by adding air circulation to the outside of the bag, you can finish the job in less than a week, though it will depend on the amount of moisture in the harvest as well as in the air.

Drying with food dehydrators

A lot of tomato growers dehydrate their crop for convenient storage. These dehydrators are great for drying Autoflowering *Cannabis*, provided you do not use the heat setting. Many dehydrators have a control switch for this. If not, don't use it. It will cook your harvest, and it will not be any good.

Again, make sure not to rush. Again, if you do, your harvest will continue to hold some of that chlorophyll you are trying to degrade. I advise use of a dehydrator for harvests only after you learn how the crop reacts to simply hanging or bag drying.

MANICURING OR TRIMMING

Once dried, you need to further clean up your harvest. This is done by carefully removing the remaining leaves, branches, and stems. Leave the tiny bract leaves and perhaps the sugar leaves right below the flowers.

Actually, most harvests undergo two manicuring sessions. First, after you harvest flowers but before you dry them, the large leaves that don't hold trichomes can be removed. Do this first trimming within 24 hours of cutting the limb. This way the leaf cells in the leaves you want to cut will still have turgor—the fan leaves will stick

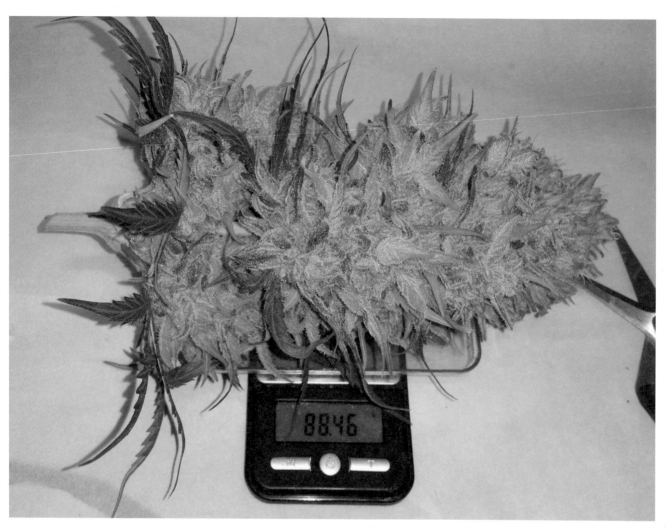

▲ After drying, you need to manicure your crop, that is, trim off all the leaves except those coated with trichomes, as in this pretty trimmed cola. GBD/DAZ MEPHISTO.

out, and they will be easier to hold and cut without damaging the trichomes.

The second trimming is after the crop dries. Remove all the small leaves. To do so, use a very fine pair of nail scissors. It is important to remember to avoid touching and thus damaging the trichomes. These are like little balloons, and they are very easy to pop open. If you must hold them, do so in your palm, not between thumb and index finger. This is an art.

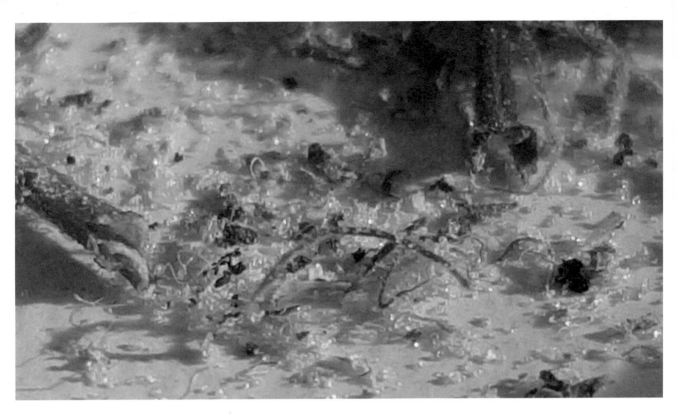

▲ Trichomes lost due to poor handing during manicuring. You don't want to lose trichomes while harvesting and trimming. *CANNABIS* PICTURES.

Your plants' flowers will be sticky. You might want to wear gloves as it is very difficult to wash off any residue. The flowers will also have a distinct odor which will increase whenever you break open trichomes while cleaning your flowers. There are special soaps that will help clean hands (and equipment).

CURING

After you dry your product, you can use it. However, it is best to take one more step, curing. The dried *Cannabis* is further dried and any remaining chlorophyll is degraded. Curing improves taste and is a step you should follow. It is not difficult. It may be what distinguishes your crop from commercial products as few commercial retailers have the time to cure properly.

To cure your harvest, carefully place it into sealable glass jars. When filling jars, do not pack or in any way smash your harvest. Instead, pour in enough to almost fill the jar and then seal it. You should be able to see the dried buds move around when you shake the jar.

Close and store jars in a cool location, out of direct sunlight, where you will have access for the first 2 weeks. If possible, open the jar up to 3 or 4 times a day to burp it, letting any gas buildup escape. Then close and shake it very gently.

After a week of daily burping, most of the chlorophyll dissipates. You can skip a day or two if you must but do check your jars regularly.

After 2 weeks or so, you can open the jars every few days. Eventually the jars won't produce gas when opened. This is the indication that the harvest is finally cured. You can see why most commercial operations don't do this. It's a lot of effort, and it takes 4 to 8 weeks. However, this effort is well worth it in terms of taste. And, if you decide it isn't, then you can skip it to future harvests. It is your hobby.

STORAGE

One of the unfortunate characteristics of Autoflowering *Cannabis* is that it becomes much less psychoactive when it is exposed to bright light and oxygen in the air. As such, it is important to store your harvest where this deterioration is minimized. The recommendation is a cool, dark location and always in a glass container.

There are now humidity control packs designed specifically to keep *Cannabis* at the right moisture level once dried and cured. Developed to keep cigars and pipe tobacco moist, they resemble sugar packs and can be placed into a jar where it will keep the moisture at a constant level. They are often sold at dispensaries and will surely be found at tobacco stores, or they can be ordered via the Internet.

Some growers vacuum pack their harvest. These packs can be kept for a long time provided that they are kept cool and in the dark. The only possible problem is the degradation of the plastic by terpenes. I do not suggest that you keep vacuum packs in the freezer as the THC will continue to degrade and trichomes will become damaged as they turn into ice crystals.

Of course, once you know how easy it is to grow Autoflowering *Cannabis*, there may be no reason to save a harvest. Simply grow a new one.

7

ENJOY YOUR HARVEST

THERE ARE LOTS of ways to use your Autoflowering *Cannabis* harvest once it has been cured. You may think smoking is the only method to ingest *Cannabis*, but never underestimate what someone who has used *Cannabis* can invent to improve the experience. (Someone said being high on *Cannabis* is the Mother of Invention.)

If you are new to *Cannabis,* you need to learn these methods. If you are returning to *Cannabis* from long ago, you will be amazed at how things have changed. Hopefully, you will be pleasantly surprised.

DECARBOXYLATION

This is absolutely key: There is an extra ring of molecules on THCA that has to be removed in order for cannabinoids to be effective. This process is known as decarboxylation and occurs when THCA is heated to 105°C (220°F). You must decarboxylate Autoflowering *Cannabis* for it to become chemically available, that is, to turn the THCA into THC. It is not hard. In fact, under some methods it is automatic.

Dry heat

The most common method of decarboxylating *Cannabis* is with heat. Heating *Cannabis* to 154°C (310°F) for 7 minutes will completely decarboxylate it. Lower temperatures work but require more time. However, lower temperatures do preserve more of the terpenes. Some suggest heating for 35 to 45 minutes at a temperature of 105°C.

Beware that if you cook at temperatures above 149°C (300°F), both the cannabinoids and the terpenes will degrade and have less of an impact. In fact, THC boils at 156.6°C (314°F).

The easiest way to decarboxylate with heat is in an oven. Preheat it to 105–115°C (220–240°F). While it warms, line a cookie tray with parchment and spread the harvest out so all of the material is heated at the same time and the same temperature. Bake away for 30 to 45 minutes.

Heating with oil

Using a slow cooker is another way to decarboxylate your Autoflowering *Cannabis* harvests. This is great for making salves. Add the dried harvest to any kind of cooking oil or lecithin, depending on the recipe. Since you do not want to overheat, determine the proper temperature using water and a thermometer. In general, 4 to 6 hours at the low setting should work. Easy.

You can also use your stovetop burner. Place equal parts cooking oil and harvest in a thick pot such as a Dutch oven or a ceramic pot. This method requires simmering, and some people add a few cups of water with every cup of oil so monitoring the temperature is easier— water boiling at a very slow simmer should be the right temperature. In addition, since the chlorophyll and herb-tasting terpenes are water soluble, they will bind to the water and not the final product.

After decarboxylation in a slow cooker or on a stove top, strain your product through cheesecloth. If you used an oil that solidifies, next place the mix in the refrigerator. Once hardened, you can lift it out of the water. If you use an oil that stays liquid at room temperature, you must wait until the water separates into its own layer and then use a spoon to retrieve the oil.

Finally, strain as many times as you want to remove as much of the particulate matter as possible. How much remains will be

THC-A	220F	strong sedative, anticonvulant
CBD-A	248F	anti-inflammatory & anti-tumor
a-Pinene	311F	anti-inflammatory, treatment of asthma
THC	315F	psychoactive; treats tumors, ADHD, nausea, & pain
Caryophyllene	349F	treats gastric reflex, depression, & anxiety
Myrcene	334F	anti-tumor, anti-inflammatory
D-Limonene	349F	treats gastric reflex, depression, & anxiety
CBD	356F	non-psychoactive; treats MS & epileptic seizures
CBN	365F	non-psychoactive; treats inflammation, tumors, insomnia
Linalool	388F	sleep aid, treats psychosis, anxiety, pain
Humulene	388F	anti-tumor, anti-inflammatory, suppresses appetite
Combustion	451F	fire releases toxic chemical by-products

determined, for the most part, by how you finely you grind the *Cannabis* before decarboxylating it.

Smoking and vaporizing

Smoking and vaporizing temperatures automatically result in decarboxylation. You do not have to treat your harvest in any way other than drying if these are the methods you use to ingest the *Cannabis.* There are all manner of devices and implements for smoking. There are many flower vaporizers on the market.

Smoking—Smoking is the most common method of ingesting *Cannabis.* It is the most obvious and so well-known that not much else need be said. It involves burning *Cannabis* in all the ways tobacco is used—pipes, water pipes, chillums, cigarettes, blunts, and so many more ways. Clearly the process decarboxylates the product.

Vaporizing—There are two forms of vaporizing Autoflowering *Cannabis.* First, there are lots of commercial *Cannabis* oil products

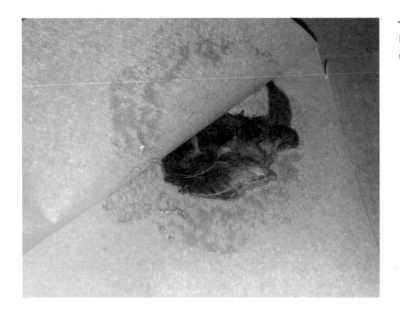

◀ Rosin from pressing flowers between wax papers. GDB/DAZ MEPHISTO.

produced by washing and soaking *Cannabis* with various gases such as carbon dioxide and butane. These result in oils with high concentrations of cannabinoids. Making these are beyond the purview of the amateur gardener. Methods of using these products are known as vaporizing.

There is another form of vaporizing which more and more *Cannabis* connoisseurs are employing. This involves heating the dried flowers just short of actual combustion, to bring the various acids such as THCA and CBDA to a boiling point. When each hits their boiling points, they change to vapors that can be inhaled. Different temperatures result in the release of different compounds, and modern commercial vaporizing instruments can be set to specific temperatures.

Rosins

Home gardeners can make an oil called "rosin" by pressing flowers. There are now commercial presses that squeeze the rosin from flowers, but these may be too expensive. All that is needed are an electric hair straightener; parchment paper; if possible, an inexpensive digital temperature gun (these infrared thermometers are available via the Internet and at art hobby stores); and a ratchet or trigger clamp.

Place small pieces of fresh (not dried) flowers in folded parchment, leaving enough room for the rosin to ooze out of the flower and still be held on the parchment. Heat the parchment packet to between 85–104°C (185–220°F) in the hair straightener.

Under extreme pressure and with a bit of heat, the chemical compounds in the flower are squeezed out onto wax paper from which they are then collected for consumption by vaporizing or even smoking.

This is where the clamp comes in: use it to very slowly put pressure on the blades of the hair straightener while the flowers heat up. Aim the heat sensor of the temperature gun on the blades to get a heat reading. If you don't have one, just observe and you will see the oils oozing out when the temperature is right.

Tinctures

Tinctures made by immersing plant materials in alcohol are an excellent way to create a stable long-term extraction of medicinals. If your intention is to include THC in a *Cannabis* extraction, then dry heat decarboxylation is necessary prior to starting any recipe. The harvest is placed in a jar and covered with a relatively high-proof alcohol of choice, then stored in a cool dark place for, say, two weeks to a year. Then it is strained, stored, and typically served for use from a dropper bottle.

There is a whole industry developing to manufacture and sell tinctures and salves. Tinctures are ingested. Salves are rubbed on the body. You can make your own both with your harvest and using the remnants of flower vaporizing, which will still contain active compounds. Various bases are used, ranging from coconut oil and emu oil for salves to grain alcohol, vodka, tequila, or brandy for tinctures.

Edibles

Eating *Cannabis,* or foods made with it, is a very popular method of using your harvest. It takes longer for the cannabinoids to take effect, but the effects last longer, often considerably longer. You can pretty much use any cooking recipe and add ground flower or use *Cannabis* infused oils.

The first key to edibles is decarboxylation, which should take place while cooking. The second is a cautious approach. Go easy, eat less than you think you need. Figure out how strong your harvests are so you can try to standardize things.

Canna butter—*Cannabis* is fat soluble, so *Cannabis* infused butter is a great way to prepare *Cannabis* for eating. It can be used in any recipe that calls for butter, everything from Bullet Coffee to Brownies. There are lots of variations. You need to test it so you will know how strong yours is and how much to use for psychoactivity.

STOVETOP CANNA BUTTER

1. Mix the *Cannabis* and the butter, add to a saucepan with the water, and bring up to a simmer, stirring to mix things. Keep on low simmer for at least 3 hours, and preferably up to 12 hours.
2. Strain and refrigerate.
3. Separate from the water after the butter solidifies.

> 18 to 30 grams *Cannabis,* finely ground
> 1 liter of water
> 250g of organic butter

CROCK-POT CANNA BUTTER

1. Mix ingredients and cook at low temp for 3 hours. Cool and separate as above.

CANNA BUTTER CHOCOLATE MUG CAKE

4 tablespoons white flour
4 tablespoons sugar
2 tablespoon cocoa
1 egg
1 to 2 tablespoons regular or bittersweet chocolate chips. Marshmallows or any berry, optional

This is a great example of how to use canna butter.
Enough canna butter for an individual

1. Microwave the mix for about 4 minutes and enjoy!

Infused Milk—Another fat-soluble product is milk, and infused *Cannabis* milk is also a great thing to have on hand for use with other items.

BASIC INFUSED MILK

0.5–1.0 gram *Cannabis*, finely ground
1 liter or quart of milk

1. Mix milk and *Cannabis* in a double boiler, or in a steel bowl placed in a cooking pot filled with water.
2. Simmer and maintain at the lowest heat for 3 hours.
3. Strain, preferably through a few layers of cheesecloth.

CANNABIS MILK SHAKE

Use infused milk with any recipe for a milkshake.

Cannabis Infused Coffee or Green Tea—Green tea and coffee make great carriers for *Cannabis*.

GREEN TEA

1. A few tablespoons of infused *Cannabis* milk and green tea.
2. Add a few drops of vanilla or peppermint.

CANNABIS COFFEE

1. A few tablespoons infused *Cannabis* milk or butter with coffee.
2. Add a few drops of vanilla or chocolate.

CANNABIS SYRUP

Cannabis syrup is a great way to add *Cannabis* to drinks or to put on anything that requires a sugary taste. Talk about a lovin' spoonful of medicine!

1. Melt the sugar into the water, add *Cannabis*, and boil for 20 minutes, ensuring that the *Cannabis* does not burn. Reduce to simmer and add glycerin for 5 minutes, stirring occasionally. Strain through several layers of cheesecloth. Use cautiously until you know its strength!

> 470 ml (3 cups US) water
> 235 ml (2 cups) sugar
> 30 ml (2 tbsp) vegetable glycerin
> 2 grams *Cannabis*, finely chopped

Firecrackers—This is a popular recipe item with lots of variations, which are all discoverable on the Internet. Firecrackers can be stored in a cookie tin and consumed at a later date.

TOASTER OVEN OR REGULAR OVEN FIRECRACKERS

Set temp at 110–120°C
(230–250°F)
0.2 to 0.5 gram *Cannabis*
(0.2 gram makes 3 to
6 sandwiches)
Saltine, Ritz, Graham, or
similar crackers
Aluminum foil
Nutella (almond or peanut
butter are suitable
substitutes)

1. Wrap *Cannabis* in the foil (like *a* Hershey's Kiss).
2. Bake for 15 minutes in aluminum foil.
3. Mix with the nut butter and put a thin layer on crackers.
4. Wrap the sandwich in foil and heat again for 15 minutes.

MICROWAVE OVEN FIRECRACKERS #1

0.2 to 0.5 gram *Cannabis*.

1. Heat the nut butter for 45 seconds on the highest setting (adding an equal amount of butter is optional).
2. Mix in *Cannabis*.
3. Wrap in foil to keep warm.
4. Eat after 15 minutes.

MICROWAVE OVEN FIRECRACKERS #2

1. Mix the nut butter, regular butter, and *Cannabis*.
2. Spread on top of crackers.
3. Microwave for 30 seconds. Some prefer bursts of several seconds. Let cool and consume.

0.2 to 0.5 gram *Cannabis*

COCONUT CANNA SPREAD

1. Mix equal parts of the ingredients.
2. Heat the mixture in a frying pan for a few minutes.

Coconut oil
Cannabis, finely ground
Powdered sugar
Vanilla

HAVE FUN, BE SAFE

Enjoy your harvest. However, be safe. When eating *Cannabis* the effects can be delayed for 2 or 3 hours. Use moderation at all times. And, by all means, respect local laws.

8

HOW TO CREATE YOUR OWN HEIRLOOM VARIETIES

ONE OF THE great things about growing tomatoes as a hobby is the ability to get as deep into it as you want. It just depends on what you want out of your hobby. So too with Autoflowering *Cannabis*.

There is a complete spectrum of activity intensity from plunking seed into soil and walking away, satisfied with only a small harvest, to developing your own heirloom seeds or clones and going for maximum yields and strength. Autoflowering *Cannabis* plants are great hobby plants.

The choice is obviously yours. However, even if you decide you are not interested in this more advanced aspect of growing Autoflowering *Cannabis*, it is a good idea to know how your Autoflowering *Cannabis* plants came to be. You might later decide this is an aspect of gardening with Autoflowering *Cannabis* that you actually would enjoy.

BREEDING FOR SEEDS

With tomatoes, breeding is pretty easy. You choose open-pollinated fruits with the best taste or size or take seed from plants that resist mildew and repeat season after season until you are satisfied. Sometimes you might paint a bit of pollen from one flower to another and come up with an interesting cross. It is pretty easy.

Autoflowering *Cannabis* plants don't have the same kind of flowers as do tomatoes. Tomatoes have one flower that has both the male and female parts. *Cannabis* produces male and female flowers. Crossing them is different.

There are a few new terms you will want to know before you begin breeding Autoflowering *Cannabis*. As with many things in the *Cannabis* world, some terms have come to be used in particular ways.

PHENOTYPES

A phenotype is the sum of the traits you see in a plant. In the Autoflowering *Cannabis* world, the word phenotype is used to describe a characteristic like height, as in tall or short phenotypes, or bushy and tree-like phenotypes. Some of these characteristics result from genetics, but others are as a result of abiotic (environmental) influences such as sunlight or temperature.

Some varieties are not stable, and so the same plants grown in the same area may be totally different phenotypes. They display different traits even though they are of the same variety. These seeds are unpredictable.

The job of the breeder is to select traits and breed them into (or out of) what will hopefully become a new wanted strain of Autoflowering *Cannabis* that is stable. This is usually accomplished by exploring traits of various available stock.

CROSSING AND BACK-CROSSING

Discovering new phenotypes with new traits can be accomplished by "crossing" two plants and then crossing the offspring with each other and seeing what appears. Or you may want to keep the trait the first cross created. This is what makes the hobby so interesting. There are so many possible outcomes.

Performing a backcross consists of breeding one of the new offspring with one of the parent plants. It stands to reason that when you perform a backcross, you end up increasing the chances the next generation will have traits like the original plant. This is because there is more genetic material identical to that of the original plant. And, it turns out, with *Cannabis* you only need to do a backcross once or twice to see results.

Of course, once you have a plant with the traits you want, you have to make sure it is stable. This can usually be accomplished by backcrossing again, one more time. This isn't as much difficult as it is time-consuming. In addition, you might not find what you are looking for or you could lose it altogether. This is why breeding Autoflowering *Cannabis* is an interesting hobby.

REALLY SIMPLIFIED GENETICS

There are lots and lots of books on genetics, and some, no doubt, were written with *Cannabis* in mind. The subject is lightly (very lightly) covered here as it is a good idea to have a picture in your mind of how Autoflowering *Cannabis* varieties come to be.

First, Autoflowering *Cannabis* is a diploid plant. This just means it gets its genes from its mother and from its father. Some genes are dominant, and some are recessive and hide in the background. Depending on the parents, different traits manifest themselves.

Since we are dealing with Autoflowering *Cannabis*, autoflowering is an important trait. By way of an extremely simple example, let's make a plant with a dominant photoperiod (P) trait and a non-photoperiod recessive trait (r).

Let's assume that the father plant has two of the P traits in its genetics, PP. The mother has two r or non-photoperiod traits, rr. (These pairs are considered homozygous for those who do crossword puzzles.)

Now, cross these homozygous plants. The father can only give a P gene to offspring. Likewise, the mother can only give an r. Thus, the offspring have one trait carrier from each parent, represented as either Pr or rP.

The fact that these first-generation crosses have two different traits makes them (in breeder speak) F1 hybrids because they are the first of the new generation made from a cross. However, if both the parents are PP, the offspring will also be PP. This is known as breeding true or true breeding.

Let's run through the possible combinations when we cross a hybrid pair, Pr with Pr. The possible combinations of offspring are PP, Pr, rP, and rr. Only the PP will be a true breeder, always creating an autoflowering offspring. The Pr and rP are hybrids that will be autoflowering because of the dominant P. Finally, the rr will be dependent on a photoperiod.

This is basic Mendelian genetics. It is not complicated, but unfortunately, while it is useful for explanations, it is not accurate. Traits are carried on DNA, and there is nothing singular about them as Mendel thought (and most of us were taught).

A few things become obvious. For example, crossing a true Autoflowering *Cannabis* with another true Autoflowering plant is easiest. In fact, it is very easy from a genetic standpoint. The day-neutral gene is recessive, but in both parents, so the possibilities of getting an rr, to keep to the simplified example, are greater.

Mixing an Autoflowering *Cannabis* with a photoperiod plant is much more difficult because the day-neutral gene is recessive. Not very many, if any, of the F1 generation from such a mix will have day-neutral traits. Statistically, the next generation will have 25% day-neutral plants, however.

Since it takes a couple of months to grow plants, you can see how breeding for a stable plant takes time. In fact, if you are lucky and all things go right, you are going to have to grow up to 6 or 7 generations before you can know your phenotype is stable and be certain that it will stay that way.

This is all a bit of work. This doesn't mean you cannot use the harvests from your female crosses if you want. And, you are not dealing with the longer growth period of regular *Cannabis*. It is even probably quicker to develop your own variety of Autoflowering *Cannabis* than your own heirloom tomato.

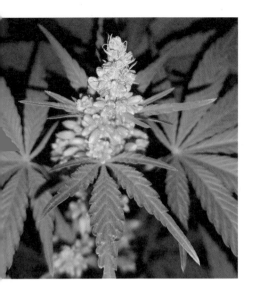

▲ A predominately male flower with some female parts. GBD/DAZ MEPHISTO.

F1 HYBRIDS AND HYBRID VIGOR

Sometimes when you cross two plants, you get a plant that does exceptionally well. This F1 hybrid is said to have hybrid vigor. If you happen to have an F1 cross that performs just as you want it, then you preserve it by recreating its lineage, not by crossing it with itself or its parent.

You should be familiar with this concept as a tomato grower. Open-pollinated seeds you can cross and recross with other open pollinated seeds. Try to breed an F1 hybrid with the same F1 hybrid, and you will not be able to maintain the so-called hybrid vigor.

The way around this is to keep a line of the parent plants going. This way you can continually recreate the cross. This is how it is done for many home garden and agricultural seeds (especially corn). It is easy to see why there is a need for professional breeders.

CHOOSING PARTNERS

Just a bit more before you know enough to start breeding (or decide to skip it and just buy seed). First, you need to choose a female partner that has the flower traits you want. This is easy as you almost always see these traits expressed because the female has flowers.

What contribution a male plant can bring to the table is a whole other matter. It is only by experimentation that you can figure out what a male plant is contributing. Once you find one capable of passing on desirable traits, you may want to stick with it for a while. It can be a time-consuming and frustrating process to cross male plants with female plants looking for desirable male traits to be passed on.

You will be pollinating one female plant with pollen from a male plant. There is some argument about pollinating feminized seed-grown females. Doing so increases the potential of getting plants that produce male and female. Just be aware. You will have to use what you have to use!

HOW TO MAKE FEMINIZED SEED

It makes sense to buy female seeds because it takes the guesswork out of growing plants that will actually develop useable buds (which males won't). Buying is also easier than creating your own feminized seeds, accomplished by forcing the female plant to produce pollen sacs.

The feminization process is started by spraying plants with colloidal silver or a growth hormone, gibberellic acid. Both of these chemicals induce female plants to produce pollen sacs at bud sites. (Untreated buds will develop into flowers, and you will see the difference.) After two weeks or so of forming, the pollen sac will swell and start to open. Keep spraying the flower up until this point.

The sac, or the leaf protecting it, will next start to open. This is when you want to collect the pollen. Too early and you may find an empty sac. (This would be a shame after all your work.) Once filled, collect the sacs with a tweezer and put them in a baggie. Shake it and the pollen will fall from the sacs. Then you collect the pollen.

Use this pollen to fertilize a female flower that is a week or so old. Obviously, this won't be from the original plant from which the seeds were developed, and this is just fine. You will be increasing genetic diversity whereas normally the plant would self-pollinate.

After a few more weeks, the fertilized calyxes will break open as seeds pop out. Congratulations. You can now plant these seeds and see what you have developed.

ASSESSING THE CHOICES

Fortunately, there are more and more breeders selling seeds of Autoflowering *Cannabis*, primarily through dispensaries, but also via the Internet in places where it is legal to ship them at this point in time. Since all of these started with the same breeding stock, it is not unusual to find crosses with the major *Cannabis indica* and *Cannabis sativa* strains.

If you are entering a breeding program, you can use already developed Autoflowering stock for your crosses, or you can use the

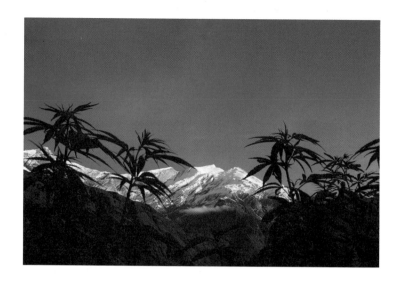

bigger cousin plants to breed with a particular Autoflowering *Cannabis* that is of interest to you.

Landraces

A landrace, or landrace variety, is a particular strain of any plant that has been developed in one specific area of the world over a period of a hundred years or more. They have always been great for breeding purposes because, having gone generation after generation without crossing with other strains, their genetics, and thus their traits, are extremely stable and don't vary among plants. They are almost invariably 100 percent *sativa* or *indica*.

With the exception of landraces, all of the thousands of varieties that are available today have been breed for special characteristics—mostly related to prohibition! There is nothing wrong with this, but for example, parents that required long growing seasons were then bred for shorter growing season length.

With legalization, plants don't have to be hidden and information about genetics can be openly exchanged. Many of the earlier desired traits no longer matter. Now breeders are going back to landraces to look for genetics from these original varieties.

These special varieties are the basis of many breeding programs. This is important because when you see the name of a country or a region in the name of a *Cannabis* strain, it is most likely a landrace (or a very close descendant of one).

Famous landraces such as Acapulco Gold and Panama Red are well-known *sativas*. Perhaps the best-known landrace *indica* is Hindu Kush. These and other landrace strains are covered in the next chapter.

My friend Tom Alexander convinced me that Autoflowering *Cannabis* plants have great landscaping potential. Tom published an early information newsletter called Sinsemilla Tips which taught many how to grow and later published a cutting-edge magazine called *Growing Edge*.

Strains for color

One of the goals of a breeding program is often to achieve various colors in the plants. Some flavonoids are yellow. Anthocyanins are red flavonoids. There are a few hundred of these pigment molecules that impart a range of blue to purple colors. Developing these is one of the goals you might want to incorporate into your own breeding program.

Tom put a few Autoflowers outdoors by a swimming pool, and they were stunning. Sure enough, these plants are quite the conversation starters. In Alaska, where we have cooler evenings, I have had plants turn a lovely purple color that only enhanced their uniqueness and delicate beauty.

More and more breeders like New Breed Seed and Mephisto are working on developing colorful plants—both flowers and leaves. Recently, I saw a plant grown from Australian seed that didn't even look like a Cannabis and, while only 10 inches tall, had hundreds of nodes. Now that prohibition is over, there will be no stopping progress!

There is an amazing array of colors to choose from to start a breeding program, since colorful photoperiod *Cannabis* flowers are great sellers in dispensaries, and commercial breeders have hunted for, and incorporated, all the colors of the rainbow. When you grow a plant with blue, yellow, purple, and pink hues, some of which scream with psychedelic overtones, you have really reached a peak in this hobby. You may not want to use it after you harvest it, as it is so pretty!

Autoflowering *Cannabis* can act like maple trees that turn color. Cool temperatures result in the stronger chlorophyll pigment

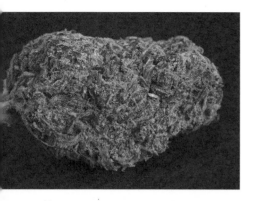

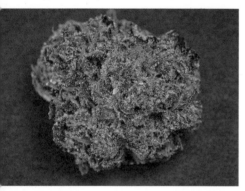

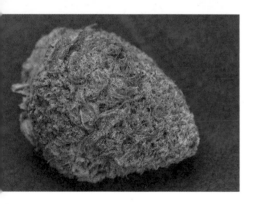

▲ The colors available for breeding are truly stunning. ADOBESTOCKPHOTOS.

breaking down and the background colors appear. Breeding stock for this kind of color change includes such famous *Cannabis* varieties as Fruity Pebbles, Black Tuna, and Pink Flower Shaman.

There are really two ways to get colorful plants. The first is to grow at least the maturing stages in cool conditions. Outdoors you are at the mercy of the climate, but indoors, it doesn't take much to provide, especially for the smaller Autoflowers, a cool environment.

Of course, achieving a cross with fantastic color may not result in a cross you want in terms of its cannabinoid content, or its flavonoids for that matter. Still, some growers won't care, just as they really don't care if that chocolate or plum tomato tastes good, just as long as it looks great.

Red and pink—Red and pink hues can be found when the pistils of some strains turn purple. Often this is caused by a lack of phosphorus, so be careful. (This is not how you want to gain the desired color.) In some varieties, it is the leaves that turn into the red zone. This is usually driven by genetics and not weather. Try any of the "Pink" named phenotypes such as Pink Lady Kush, Pink Lemonade, or Pink Flower Shaman.

Yellow hues—Yellow colors are caused by carotenoids and flavonoids just like in vegetables and fruits. The flowers display the color. They are induced by cold temperatures, too, when the green chlorophyll fades, but also by alkaline conditions.

Alien OG, Grapefruit, Lemon Kush (Lemon! How appropriate), Kandy, Skunk, and Wicked OG can display yellows. Yellow varieties often have gold as part of their names. (Acapulco Gold, anyone?)

Black hues—Black is not really the color displayed, but it is the right term for what is a whole range of dark flower colors that are close to black. If the genetics are there, cold (10°C, 50°F) temperatures can induce leaves to show a dark color (but that is very cool, at least for the vegetative stage).

There are some strains that don't require weather to display color. These phenotypes often have black in their names: Black Diesel, Black Mamba, Black Willy, Black Widow, Black Tuna, and a landrace, Vietnamese Black. Violetta and Malawi can be used as well. These have dark purple leaves by the time of harvest.

Strains for THC

Obviously, one might want to develop a high THC producing strain. This is the major cannabinoid that is measured by labs, as it has been (wrongly) assumed to be the only thing that controls the plant's psychoactivity. Look for numbers of 20% THC or higher.

Current high (sorry) percentages for THC have just started to reach over 30% of the plant's resin, as of this printing. This is a great increase over earlier years and are a direct result of breeding programs.

Strains for CBD

CBD does not produce a psychoactive response, as you now know. It impacts the body but not the brain. It is in great demand by those who want some of the plant's medical benefits, however. During prohibition days, no one paid much attention to CBD, so there wasn't much effort to increase its numbers. Things have changed. Now there are 100 % CBD strains, even in the Autoflowering arena.

SEED STORAGE

If you grow your own seed, you are going to end up with more seeds than you can possibly plant. This is both because these little plants can produce a lot of seed when you let them, but also because you are probably limited in how many plants you are allowed to grow, unless you are a licensed commercial or caregiver grower. Store excess seeds in an airtight container in a dark, cool spot or give them away!

Fortunately, *Cannabis* seeds can be stored for 5 or 6 years before they begin to deteriorate. Light, temperature, and moisture are key things to control. You also need to protect your seeds from pests like

I accidently discovered some purple Autoflowering *Cannabis* one fall when Alaskan cold temperatures hit my plants, destroying chlorophyll and leaving purple anthocyanidins. One or two weeks of exposure at 7–10°C (45–50°F) will do the trick. Over 14°C (75°F) the chlorophyll returns.

rodents and birds (*Cannabis* seed, in the form of hemp, is in bird feed mixes), as well as from ethylene exposure.

You will need a glass container for storage. These do not leak. Plastic baggies are not the way to go as they often are not airtight and deteriorate. (Especially in the presence of piney-smelling Autoflowering *Cannabis*, right?) Do not forget to label your jar.

It is imperative that seed goes into storage dry and remains dry. To ensure this, you will need to end up with seeds that have about 2 to 4 percent water. Use a desiccant pack to absorb the moisture in the jar and hold it. These have the added advantage of absorbing the small amounts of ethylene given off by the seeds, which has a deleterious effect on them.

Some freeze seeds to store them, but that is not a suggestion I support. Instead, a cold room, a basement, a crawl space, or a garage will do. You can use the refrigerator, of course, and this may be the easiest, but you have to worry about fluctuations in temperature. (Place your jars way in the back and don't open the door so much!) A dedicated refrigerator may be called for, depending on how deep you get into breeding. (However, even leftover seeds from a packet should be stored properly.)

It is light, temperature, and humidity fluctuations that should be avoided. This is why it might make sense to keep your seeds in a jar in a dark room that maintains temperature, instead of a refrigerator that is in constant use. It is up to you.

CLONING AUTOFLOWERING *CANNABIS* IS NOT PRACTICAL

Traditionally, cloning (simply growing a plant from cuttings) has not been a method for reproducing Autoflowering *Cannabis*. One reason for this has to do with the size of the early Autoflowering *Cannabis* plants. These were originally really small, about 12 inches. It was, frankly, pretty hard to take a viable cutting which would have enough nodes to work with.

In addition, Autoflowering *Cannabis* plants simply grow too fast for cuttings to root and develop a worthwhile number of flowers. Super Autoflowering *Cannabis* plants may have long enough branches and take longer to grow. If you want to try cloning, use these and take cuttings early.

The best time to take a cutting to use as a clone is around the 3rd week. As you now know, for many Autoflowers, this is simply too late. Flowers will have appeared. You are really wasting your time if a clone is taken too long after the first white pistils appear.

If you do decide to try and clone, take your cuttings carefully. You want to use a sharp razor blade and cut one of the very lowest branches close to the main stem. Ideally, it should have three nodes, but you might get away with two. Remove leaves starting to grow from the bottom node of the cutting, split the stem from the bottom up 1/2 inch (give or take, depending on what you have to work with). Use a sterilized razor blade or sharp knife.

Then dip the cutting into rooting hormone, which you can get at nurseries and grow stores. Place the cutting into a small container of potting soil. Cover it with a plastic bag or similar material to make a tent, keeping in the humidity.

The clone should root in a week. It will probably be going into flower, but it will grow and develop buds. These may be a big "meh," or they may even surpass those of the mother plant. And, since this is not the normal way to reproduce your plants (although it is fun), when it works you get bragging rights in the Autoflowering *Cannabis* community and with your fellow home gardeners.

SOME FINAL TIPS

Breeding Autoflowering *Cannabis* plants is not difficult, but it does take time and so it takes patience. There are a few rules to keep in mind, and the very first is not to skimp on genetics. You should use high-quality seed to begin with. This probably means pre-feminized seeds are the only way to go, unless you are looking to produce pollen from a male plant or expand your skills in growing by getting into feminization of your own seeds.

Find seed from breeders you can trust. Seed packets should contain a lot of information and a picture, or should direct you to a website that contains information. The genetics of the strain should be listed so you can look up the variety and know what you are working with. Don't buy unless you really understand what you are getting.

If nothing else, learn to appreciate those commercial breeders who work to keep happy all those who are not interested in producing their own seeds.

9

AUTOFLOWERING BREEDING STOCK: SOME CLASSICS TO KNOW, GROW, AND USE

AN EVER-INCREASING NUMBER of commercial *Cannabis* breeders are developing Autoflowering *Cannabis* seeds for use in commercial production and also for sale to home gardeners. As a result, there are plenty of Autoflowering varieties from which to choose seed, with more coming online all the time. These are available to grow and for your own breeding program, should you decide to experiment.

For a home gardener, the seed selection process can be overwhelming, if not bewildering. (It is no different with tomato selections!) The confusion is for three reasons, not the least of which is that most gardeners do not yet have experience with various types of Autoflowering *Cannabis* plants. You gradually learned about plum, heritage, early, and other types of tomatoes. It is the same with Autoflowering *Cannabis*.

Next, there isn't a standardized system for naming varieties based on proven genetics. This allows plants to be named after such diverse things as pets, fruits, breakfast cereals, girlfriends, famous people, and all manner of locations around the world. There is even one variety named for a US president (Obama Kush).

The third reason there is confusion is because most of the varieties of seed today are either the results of efforts to grow better *Cannabis* during prohibition or the progeny of those efforts. Again, all of this breeding work was done underground because of prohibition. There was little cross communication among the community of growers and little help from universities and researchers. Nor was it possible to grow in the best places, unimpeded.

What we know now is that unless you have a DNA test done on your plants, there is no way to be sure what you are really growing. Still, there are a few ways to help make the determination as to what seeds you want to grow.

The best is to have test results. It is now possible to determine the chemical contents of *Cannabis*. Initially, tests concentrated on THC and CBD percentages. Today, there is a growing (literally) recognition that terpenes and flavonoids are also important, and many breeders are including these in their test reports. Yours will not be an exact duplicate, but what you grow should be close to what the breeder's numbers reveal.

If there are no test results available, then you should next study the plant's ancestry. The names of Autoflowering *Cannabis* varieties often mimic the names of their established and well-known larger cousins. Those selling seed almost always provide cultural information that includes an explanation of the plant's lineage. If this information is not found on the seed package, look for a website to supplement handouts at stores. (See Resources.)

The point is, if you know some of the standby, popular, big-plant *Cannabis* types, it will help in understanding what you are growing or want to grow in terms of Autoflowering *Cannabis*. This is particularly so as more and more efforts are underway to identify and use landraces now that prohibition allows for a concerted and open effort to commercialize *Cannabis*.

LANDRACE VARIETIES

Landraces have always been great for *Cannabis* breeding purposes. They are genetically stable, 100% *sativa* or 100% *indica*, and relatively rare. This made them ideal for developing new varieties. They were collected in the 1960s and '70s and are now often hoarded for commercial breeding purposes.

All of the seeds available for growing *Cannabis* today owe their genetics to approximately 40 of these landrace strains. If there is a country in the name of a *Cannabis* strain, it is most likely either a landrace or a very close descendant of one. Well-known *sativa* landrace varieties include Acapulco Gold, Durban Poison, and Panama Red. Perhaps the best-known landrace *indica* is Hindu Kush.

Knowing the landraces used for breeding is useful because each does have stable traits. Each has its own unique flavor and profile of terpenes and cannabinoids. It is worth noting a few. You will quickly become familiar with them as you get deeper into growing Autoflowers. This information will help you choose which seed varieties to grow.

Afghanistan and Pakistan landraces

Hindu Kush is the most famous of these strains, which are all *indica*. In fact, as a group they are often known as Hindu Kush. They were originally grown at high altitudes, where it is very dry, and were grown to make hashish, which demands lots and lots of trichomes. They produce profusely from small plants because they develop lots of branches.

The most famous Hindu Kush landrace is Afghani, also known as Affie or Afghani #1. It became the basis for all breeding programs because it ripens in mid-October when started in the spring. This was very early for *Cannabis* growers as most are not harvestable until December and even January.

The relatively short growing season (wow, what would an Autoflower have done for them?) meant you could grow outdoors without using a greenhouse. Hindu Kush was used for a lot of hybrids because of this. They are small and stocky plants with lots of resin production so, when you grew them clandestinely indoors, you didn't need as much space.

In addition to Hindu Kush, Lashkar Gah and Mazar i Sharif are other less well-known varieties. Progeny of breeding programs using these include Bubba Kush and Purple Afghani.

Jamaican landrace

These plants were grown from seed imported from India by workers and advisors the British brought to Jamaica to work plantations. They are all *sativas* and produce a very strong psychoactive response when used.

The famous reggae singer Bob Marley grew up in Jamaica. Lamb's Bread and King's Bread were his most beloved Caribbean landrace strains.

South American landraces

Mexico, Panama, Columbia, and many other South American countries are home to famous landraces. Some of these were developed in the mountains and others on the low plains, but all had the advantage of a great equatorial growing season. These are all *sativa* plants and were also developed from plants brought over to the Western Hemisphere by workers who first arrived in the Caribbean.

Producing a long central stem and lots of THC, but also CBD and CBNA, the most well-known South American landrace is Colombian Gold. It was an early favorite in the 60s. Less well-known, but utilized for all manner of breeding, are Cali Hills, Punto Rojo, and Santa Marta Gold. These have been used to breed Cheese, Skunk, and Haze.

African landraces

Africa has a long history of cultivating *Cannabis*. It is home to some of the most interesting landrace strains. Given the size of the continent, these can be very different.

The most famous African landraces are Malawi Gold and Durban Poison. Both plants take advantage of a long growing season. They produce tremendous amounts of resin. They are both *sativa* strains.

You may encounter Swazi Gold and Kilimanjaro, both obviously African. These are sturdy plants with buds that have elongated calyxes and very few leaves. They tend to flower for a long time and are known for producing a sweet resin.

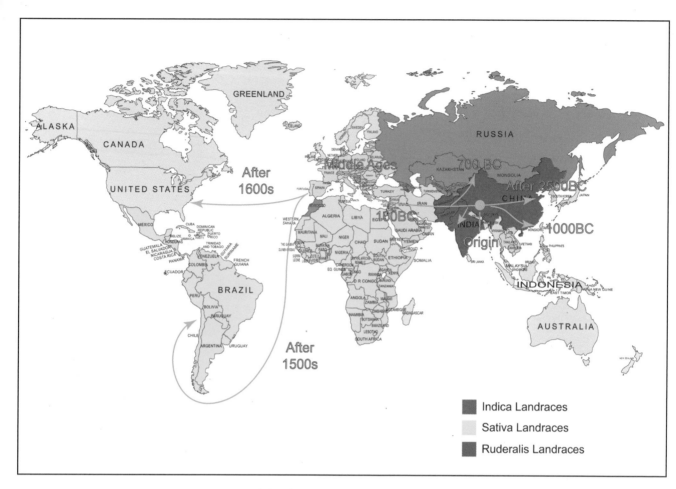

▲ Landrace map

Thai and Southeast Asian landraces

Thai landrace strains have special elongated flowers with a fantastic citrus aroma and strong psychoactive effects. Plants have high amounts of THC and low amounts of CBCA and CBD. They are all *sativa*, and the most famous are Thai, Aceh, and Chocolate Thai; and Luang Prabang from Laos.

North American landrace strains

Ever since the 60s, the search has been on for North American landrace strains. They have been found in Mexico with Acapulco Gold, and there is a Hawaiian strain known as Maui Wowie.

Miscellaneous strains

There is a landrace strain for every region. It doesn't matter if you are in Morocco, Lebanon, Russia, or Pakistan, there is most probably at least one landrace variety worthy of including in a breeding program. Again, you should note the presence of countries in names, as this is the big tip-off that you have a strain with landrace ancestors.

TEN CLASSIC VARIETIES

In addition to pure landraces, there are some modern bred varieties that have enough cachet to be famous. These are sought-after and are the basis of many commercial breeding programs.

The home gardener should recognize some of the very well-known varieties sold in dispensaries and used for breeding purposes. When you see the names of these in the variety or its lineage, they indicate unique characteristics. Look for them.

Haze

This one has to be on the top of most lists. According to friend George Van Patten, aka Jorge Cervantes, it is found in the genetics of 10 to 15 percent of all *Cannabis*. This *sativa* was developed in the 1960s and '70s in Santa Cruz, California, and is said to have Colombian, Mexican, Thai, and Indian *sativa* in its genes. These are all narrow-leaf *sativa* varieties. The plant is known for its pine and lemon tastes and is at once both sweet and spicy.

The buds of Haze plants are thin, so it does not make a good cross for bud size; look for other advantages, like its disease resistance and the long period before it produces seeds, which could make some of its genes useful when you want to develop a strain you can clone.

Look for Super Silver Haze and Lemon Haze, two famous off-breeds using Haze genetics. They show what breeding can do for a varietal strain.

Hindu Kush

Hindu Kush can produce some very strong psychoactivity. This is a true Kush, meaning it was originally developed for use as a hash plant. The flowers were meant to be dried and sifted to recover the trichomes. It is an Afghani *indica* that dates back to at least the 13th century.

The harvest from these plants tends to impart a very sedative effect. The taste is often described as harsh or raw. This is because these plants were really originally bred for producing hash.

Skunk

Skunk? What kind or name is that for something that you might ingest? Still, a lot of Dutch-produced seeds have this in their genes, and Cervantes suggests that 30% of all *Cannabis* has this strain in their genes. When it was developed and released, it was like a revolution in the world of *Cannabis* breeding.

It is hard to believe, but Skunk actually tastes sweet. It is *sativa* and produces a very strong "head" high. It has a lot of both Columbian and Acapulco Gold, which actually makes it an *indica-sativa* mix. Its colas are nice and thick, just the thing to breed into an Autoflower. And it flowers early, in usually between 50 and 70 days.

Afghan

This landrace from Afghanistan has been bred and bred ever since it was brought to the United States in the 1970s. Today, Afghan or Afghani #1 or Affie is the foundation of almost every single *indica* plant breed.

Afghan is often considered the variety that gave rise to the prohibition-era reputation of a *Cannibis* with a killer (meaning very good) stoner effect. It is strong. It has lots of myrcene and has a distinct, sedative couch-lock impact on users, as opposed to a cerebral high.

AK-47

It is unclear what the AK stands for in this variety, but it makes sense for it to be Afghan Kush. What is certain is that the name has nothing to do with the AK-47 machine gun used in Afghanistan at the time of its "discovery." That part of the name probably comes from the Dutch labeling system used during breeding development.

AK-47 is an unusual plant in that it develops phenotypes, that is, plants from the same seeds that look different. They can be either broad-leafed or narrow-leafed. Amazingly, plants can appear to be *sativa* or *indica*, depending on phenotype.

AK-47 is a mix of Thai, Afghan, and Brazilian genetics. It has a blend of myrcene and beta-caryophyllene. This gives it a split personality, as would be expected from a variety that produces so many phenotypes. It can be disorienting at times but cause the user to become focused at others.

Northern Lights

From the West Coast of Canada (some say the American Northwest), Northern Lights is an *indica-sativa* mix that became very popular in the 80s and continues to be so today. It has a very piney taste that is also sweet. It is an extremely popular strain to cross with other plants, including Autoflowering *Cannabis,* perhaps because it has northern genetics and produces quickly. Northern Lights has great yields. Better, they come after only 65 days or so.

Northern Lights has lots of pinene, as the taste reveals, but also myrcene and beta-caryophyllene. It produces an almost psychedelic and fast high—not likely to be the best experience for beginners to using *Cannabis.*

Blueberry

This is a very famous cross that really took over the *Cannabis* world for a time. Its smell is reminiscent of the blueberries that also grow in Oregon, where the strain was developed.

These plants have a nice stimulating high and a reputation for helping with appetite. They have uplift from limonene due to their Thai and Mexican genes and a bit of sedation due to the myrcene from their Afghan genes. The unusual stimulating high does not prevent one from going to sleep.

Once you start growing, you might develop a new strain and become famous. That is what happened to an Oregon gentlemen who is now a living legend in the world of *Cannabis*. His name, D.J. Short. He is responsible for developing the famous strain known as Blueberry. Apparently, the Thai sticks prevalent during the Vietnam conflict are at the base of its genetics, along with some Mexican or Acapulco Gold, and Afghan *Cannabis*.

Blueberry smells just like blueberries with a hint of spice and was crossed with Haze to produce another variety with fantastic taste and appeal, Blue Dream. In fact, there are a lot of *Cannabis* varieties with Blue in the name that derive genetics from D.J. Short's efforts, such as Azure Dream. This an example (and proof) that breeding is a never-ending process and you never know what you might develop.

Blue Dream

This is an example of using popular strains for breeding. It is a cross between Blueberry and Haze. This is a mix that makes Blue Dream both relaxing and stimulating. It also is a good example of a silly name, as there is little dreaming with this strain. It is not a couch lock *Cannabis*. It is, however, an easy to grow plant (a dream to grow?) developed in California. Blue Dream has a reputation for needing tremendous amounts of water.

OG Kush

There is a debate whether OG stands for Organically Grown or Original Grow, but according to another story, this was Kush grown near the ocean as opposed to in the mountains. Ocean Grown, hence the OG.

All manner of *Cannabis* is sold under the appellation OG. (Only genetics will reveal the truth, but at least you won't assume it stands for organic!) Regardless, OG Kush is known for being very strong and flavorful. It seems to have Afghan, Nepali, and Thai genetics.

OG Kush has an orangey, citrusy taste but not a tart one. Full of uplifting limonene and lots of myrcene as well, it is full of other terpenes, including beta-caryophyllene, linalool, and alpha-humulene. The high it imparts can be very strong, and many would say this is not a *Cannabis* for beginners.

Cannatonic

With increasing interest in CBD, breeders developed high-CBD breeds. These became all the rage after it was demonstrated on a national US news show that one plant, called Charlotte's Web, greatly improved the life of a young girl who has a severe form of seizures. A breeding frenzy ensued.

One of the most famous results of these efforts is Cannatonic, a *Cannabis* good for relaxing muscles, but usually with little THC and thus little psychoactivity. Other similar varieties include Harlequin and Granny Durkel. (Where do they come up with these names?)

AND MORE

As noted, there are always new varieties of *Cannabis* coming in to the market. Autoflowering seed variety has increased exponentially from the early days of those first Lowryders. Throughout, there has been homage paid to the early varieties of *Cannabis* that made what we have today.

As you now know, breeding Autoflowering *Cannabis* is within the reach of the home gardener, should you decide to try your hand at it. If you do breed your own, keep the important lineage in the name, or at least keep track of it. You never know where your efforts may end up!

10

THE FUTURE OF AUTOFLOWERING *CANNABIS*

I ATTENDED COLLEGE IN the 1960s. Back then, I never would have guessed that *Cannabis* would be legal anywhere, that strains could be improved, or that Autoflowering types would be developed and made available to gardeners. My early record for predictions is not very good.

Of course, back then no one really knew it was the just the flowers that contained the sought-after psychoactive (and medicinal) chemicals. Who had even heard of CBD? Heck, how cannabinoids impacted the body hadn't been discovered and wouldn't be for years.

Today, it is much easier to see the future of *Cannabis,* and Autoflowering *Cannabis* in particular, starting with my first prediction. There is no doubt in my mind that Autoflowering varieties will become more and more popular, both as plants for the home gardener as well as for use by commercial growers.

It seems pretty clear to me that there is a wonderful future for these plants. In fact, let me make a few more predictions.

AUTOFLOWERING *CANNABIS* WILL BE THE NEXT TOMATO

Autoflowering *Cannabis,* so perfect a plant for home gardeners, will become not only acceptable but popular. They really *are* going to be the next tomato, providing lots of fun and entertainment to home gardeners. Given my frequent comparisons throughout this book, you probably could have guessed this prediction.

If the past 50 years of home-growing tomatoes has shown anything, it is that once a plant becomes embedded in gardening culture, all manner of gardeners take it up. Some just grow as they have been told. Others go beyond and push on, and extend, the frontiers of what was thought possible. My second prediction is that you can expect new methods to be discovered and developed.

And if the cultivation of regular *Cannabis* over the past 50 years has shown me anything, it is that the next 50 years will result in all manner of new Autoflowering *Cannabis* varieties. Just look at the number of Autoflowering *Cannabis* varieties that already exist. One can certainly see why a hobby gardener might get excited to be able to grow them.

LANDRACE DETERMINATION AND RESULTANT USE

There will be a big movement to go back and discover *Cannabis's* roots, so to speak. Unfortunately, there is no longer easy access to many of the landrace strains as original seed stock has disappeared or is being held for private use. However, DNA detection will be used to rediscover landrace strains and their progeny, helping breeders back-cross to regain them.

Eventually, breeders won't even need the actual landrace strain itself, only the genetic sequence of it so that the best part of the plant will be included in future plants. There are already yeasts that can produce cannabinoids. What is next, I can't tell, but there is definitely a new world coming.

BETTER *CANNABIS*

Next, and here is an easy one, I predict we will have even better Autoflowering *Cannabis*. New breeding programs will track genetics out in the open, using all of the tools and skills possible. Ultimately, genome sequencing will allow us to improve all aspects of growing Autoflowering plants.

All aspects of these plants are open for improvement: visual impact, taste, and smell; and optimization of the quantities and proportions of chemicals is already within reach. Over the next 10 years, discoveries will be made to improve every aspect of the use of these plants, from growing to ingestion.

Hardiness, or heat tolerance—As we go deeper into global warming, heat tolerance will be bred into some varieties, as will the ability to do well with less water. (After we deal with global warming, cold tolerance will be worked on!) Some breeders, home gardeners included, will concentrate on the size of plants. So many other dreams of growers will come true. Who knows, a home gardener just like you may even participate in the research.

Pest resistance—Genetics will also be used to develop varieties that are resistant to specific pests and pathogens. It is hard to imagine a world without root aphids (but it was hard for this 70-year-old to imagine a world were *Cannabis* was legal). Breeders will identify plants that produce metabolites to counter pathogens like powdery mildew, for example. Resistance to various pathogens and pests will be bred into plants.

Medicine—Over the next 50 years, Autoflowering *Cannabis* will be used to develop specific medicines. We know what particular cannabinoids, flavonoids, and terpenoids do, and we are learning more every day. We are probably going to discover new compounds in Autoflowering *Cannabis*. For research purposes, these fast-growing plants are just the ticket.

We already have the ability to identify the genetics which control the production of most *Cannabis* chemicals. Over the next 50 years, this will result in the development of all manner of different Autoflowering *Cannabis* varieties, capable of meeting a wide range of medical needs. You may even be able to grow your own medicines.

Different looking plants—Again, given how things have gone in the past with other plants, there is every reason to believe that over the next 50 years there will be Autoflowering *Cannabis* plants that look different than they do today. Some will be bigger while others may even be smaller. The number of nodes on stems will be studied and optimized as well as maturation times, color, and habit.

There will be colorful or interestingly shaped Autoflowering *Cannabis* plants developed for landscaping. These will be used for annual hedges and for texture in the garden.

And, no doubt, there will be Autoflowering *Cannabis* developed for holidays. It won't just be Poinsettias, anymore. And then there is *Cannabis's* own holiday, April 20th.

STANDARDIZED NAMING

In the future there will be a better system for naming Autoflowers. There has to be one developed. Things are a mess today. Genetic testing will help, but so will a general understanding and universal acceptance of some system.

The wine industry has it right. Perhaps location, *terroir,* will take hold, at least for the outdoor grower. Perhaps it already has, since the whole concern about landrace origins is essentially a discussion of terroir. Groupings as with Pinots, Sauvignon, and the like make more sense than the hodgepodge of confusion we have now. One day, there will be an international naming convention for all *Cannabis* along with a central register to keep track of things.

EASY AVAILABILITY

Here is another easy prediction: more and more sources of Autoflowering *Cannabis* seed will become available. Now that things are legal in so many jurisdictions, you will be able to buy your own seed from seed racks just like you do tomatoes.

And, just as with tomatoes and other flowers and vegetables, there will be websites and even some paper catalogs which will

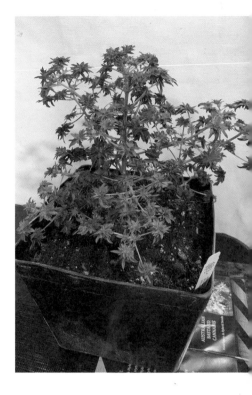

▲ Australian Bastard. Reportedly grown by an Aboriginal for at least 60 years before "discovery," this unusual looking plant is tiny with a tremendous number of nodes, making it a perfect candidate for breeding with Autoflowering *Cannabis*. JUDITH HOERSTING.

specialize in providing myriad choices of seed to the home gardener. Of course, you will also be able to find seed for sale in the existing garden web and catalog outlets, only there will be more of them and more choices in the Autoflowering *Cannabis* category.

It is even probable that nurseries and perhaps even supermarkets will sell not only Autoflowering seed but Autoflowering *Cannabis* plants in pre-flowering stages. There will be celebratory Autoflowering *Cannabis* plants for sale on 4/20 day (look it up, if you are not familiar with this date) and perhaps color-oriented plants for holidays like Christmas and Saint Patrick's Day.

Admittedly, these changes may not come fast, but that this book will be sold in many venues, where just a short while ago it was not legal to possess Autoflowering *Cannabis*, is proof that it will happen. It takes a while for a stigma caused by incessant and constant brainwashing to disappear (which is why we don't use the M word).

SPECIALIZED EQUIPMENT

As with anything in the hobby gardening arena, it doesn't take much to see there will be a great deal of improvement in specialized equipment used to grow Autoflowering *Cannabis* at home. Lights immediately come to mind.

Future lights will provide the very exact wavelengths necessary to optimize your plant's production of cannabinoids, flavonoids, and terpenoids. Home plasma bulbs the size of marbles will duplicate the sun's light.

Equipment will come in all sorts of form factors to fit any home growing situation. The latest reflector material will be utilized. Heat efficiency will be extreme, as will power efficiency.

GROWING AUTOFLOWERING
CANNABIS WILL BE EVEN EASIER

It is not hard to fathom the use of AI, Artificial Intelligence, to help grow Autoflowering *Cannabis*. It won't just be Autoflower gardeners who will benefit, but their plants, too. Receptors will be attached and will automatically water at the proper time or increase air circulation or constantly adjust temperatures.

It will be possible to automatically feed Autoflowering *Cannabis* plants the right kind of nutrient after determining the existence of a deficiency. There will even be a way to set a signal for your (and your plant's) optimal time for harvesting.

There will be special reflective tents in which to grow your plants as well. They already exist, with built-in light timers and automatic watering components. However, in the future, they will be easily controlled by computers and cell phones. You will be able to put your plants into a tent and walk away until harvest time. I predict, however, that many will forgo these automatic solutions. Using them isn't much of a hobby.

Specialty soil mixes will be developed. These will include soils with a precise mix of soil food web members to properly populate protect and feed Autoflowering *Cannabis*.

GOVERNMENT INVOLVEMENT

The crystal ball on the future role of government when it comes to *Cannabis,* and Autoflowering *Cannabis* in particular, is hazy (sorry). Much of what is regulated comes from prohibition mentality. In some instances, this comes with a big wallop of stigmatization. Hopefully, this will change. People used to think tomatoes were poisonous. Maybe growing Autoflowering *Cannabis* will help change attitudes for the better.

While it is difficult to make predictions, governmental regulations, once in place, are hard to get rid of. Tax revenues have been a big carrot in the legalization movement. These have all been predicated on the supposed sinfulness of using and growing *Cannabis*.

Given all governments' need for money, the idea that taxes gained from sales will go away is simply not realistic, and history tells us that there are going to be more of them. To be successful, however, the government will need to continue to foster the notion that there is something intrinsically wrong about growing and using that justifies the tax. I predict this will become increasingly difficult.

More realistic, and important to the hobby grower of Autoflowering *Cannabis,* will be elimination of the limitations that have been placed on the number of plants the gardener can grow at home without a license. Can you imagine being limited to growing 6 tomatoes, only 2 of which could be in flower? At some point, gardeners will unite and demand an end. Can you imagine a tax to grow a tomato plant?

PUBLIC RECOGNITION AND ACCEPTANCE

Overriding all the other predictions, once *Cannabis* is legal everywhere, gardeners around the world will be joined together by an exciting new category of plants. That is one prediction you can count on. Autoflowering *Cannabis* will, indeed, be grown by home gardeners in the exact manner we as a group grow tomatoes.

I am not so sure that too many gardeners will annoy their neighbors by leaving baskets of Autoflowering *Cannabis* harvest on door steps, but all manner of foods will be baked with the harvest of Autoflowering plants, and many will concoct homemade remedies (which is exactly what happened with photoperiod *Cannabis* in the past— back to the future, huh?).

There will be categories in various agricultural fairs with gardeners proudly competing for ribbons and proudly showing off and sharing the fruits (flowers) of their efforts.

There will be magazines, most probably web-based ezines, on growing Autoflowers. These will be full of recipes, breeding suggestions, variety developments, equipment and seed ads, and other predictable fare.

Heck, you might even learn how to make paper or rope out of your stems from a TV or YouTube show. (I can see the Martha Stewart now.) You are going to find TV and print stories about Autoflowering *Cannabis* and see them everywhere in the background *as if they were just a beautiful plant.*

IT'S A BRIGHT FUTURE

The final prediction? Without a doubt, there is a bright future for growing Autoflowering *Cannabis*. There are no limitations in growing it at home, and gardeners just like you all around the world will embrace these new plants. That is one prediction you can count on.

RESOURCES

BLOGS AND LISTSERVS

Autoflower.net
https://www.autoflower.net

The Weed Blog
https://www.weedblog.com

The Growery
https://www.growery.org

Grass City
https://www.GrassCity.com

Marijuana.com
https://www.marijuana.com

CANNABIS LOCATORS AND INFO SITES WITH VARIETAL DESCRIPTIONS

Weedmaps—will help you find the locations of dispensaries that sell seed. It will also describe strain attributes.

htpps://www.weedmaps.com

Leafly—will help you find the locations of dispensaries that sell seed. It will also describe strain attributes. There is a free newsletter.

https://www.Leafly.com

MAGAZINES

High Times—Started during the mid-1970s, this magazine was the standard for a full generation while *Cannabis* possession was illegal. It has a great website and continues its work. https://hightimes.com

Free—Print magazines come and go, but there are numerous publications available free at dispensaries.

PREMIXED ORGANIC SOILS

There are lots of premix soils. Here are some names to look for, though don't overlook local brands. It might be helpful to get recommendations at a grow store if you are new to indoor soils.

Roots Organics
ProMix BX
FoxFarm/Happy Frog
Miller Soils
Black Gold

FURTHER READING

Books by the author

A trilogy of books that explains the organic system. All are must-reads.

Teaming with Microbes: The Organic Gardener's Guide to the Soil Food Web, Timber Press, revised ed., 2011

Teaming with Nutrients: The Organic Gardener's Guide to the Optimization of Plant Nutrition, Timber Press, 2013

Teaming with Fungi: The Organic Growers Guide to Mycorrhizae, Timber Press, 2017

Books by Jorge Cervantes

George Van Patten used the alias Jorge Cervantes to write grow books during prohibition. His were some of the first to popularize home growing of *Cannabis*.

His books are published by his eponymously named publishing house, Van Patten Publishing, http://www.vanpattenpublishing.com

Marijuana Grow Basics: The Easy Guide for Cannabis Aficionados, Van Patten Publishing, 2009.

Marijuana Horticulture: The Indoor/Outdoor Medical Grower's Bible, Van Patten Publishing, 2006. There were six editions.

The Cannabis Encyclopedia, the Definitive Guide to Cultivation and Consumption of Marijuana, Van Patten Publishing, 2015. This is a revised and extended version of *Marijuana Horticulture* with more than twice the original text and a thousand more images. Foreword by Vicente Fox Quesada.

Books by Ed Rosenthal

Ed Rosenthal was an early *Cannabis* entrepreneur and pioneer in the legalization movement. He paid the price for seed development and sale during prohibition. His books are available through his website, www.edrosenthal.com

Ed Rosenthal's Marijuana Grower's Handbook

Marijuana Pest and Disease Control

Beyond Buds, Next Generation: Marijuana Concentrates and Cannabis Infusions

Other suggested books

Growing Indoors for Fun and Profit, by Michael Wolf Segal (aka Farmer in the Sky), pioneering grower and advocate of legalization. He is responsible for developing the Sea of Green method of cultivation. *Growing Indoors* was first published as a pamphlet in 1985. Limited availability.

True Living Organics: The Ultimate Guide to Growing All-Natural Marijuana Indoors, 2nd ed. 2016, by The Rev, an early organic convert who quickly became a guru to others he converted.

What Is Wrong with My Marijuana Plant? A Cannabis Grower's Visual Guide to Easy Diagnosis and Organic Remedies, paperback 2018, by David Deardorff and Kathryn Wadsworth. They have a similar book for tomatoes.

Growing Marijuana: A QuickStart Indoor / Outdoor Grower's Guide for Medical and Personal Marijuana Cultivation, 2016, by Gary Keller and R. Moore.

POPULAR SEEDBANKS

Barney's Farm

https://www.seedsupreme.com/seed-banks/barney-s-farm.html

Big Buddha Seeds

https://www.bigbuddhaseeds.com

Cali Connection

https://www.seedsupreme.com/seed-banks/cali-connection.html

DNA Genetics

https://www.seedsupreme.com/seed-banks/dna-genetics.html

Dinafem

https://www.dinafem.org/en/autoflowering-*Cannabis*-seeds/

Dutch Passion

https://www.dutch-passion.com/en/

Greenhouse Seeds

https://www.seedsupreme.com/seed-banks/green-house-company.html

Mephisto Genetics

https://www.Mephisto-genetics.html

New Breed Seed

http://www.newbreedseed.com/

Nirvana Seeds

https:www.nirvana-seeds.com

Pyramid Seeds

https://www.pyramidseeds.com/

Royal Queen Seeds

https://www.seedsupreme.com/seed-banks/royal-queen-seeds.html

Seedsman

https://www.seedsman.com

Sensi Seeds

https:www.sensi-seeds.com

Suzy Seeds

https://suzyseeds.com/*Cannabis*-seeds/autoflowering/blue-berry-fruit-auto

Seed Supreme

https://www.seedsupreme.com/seed-banks/tga-subcool-genetics.html

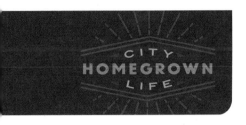

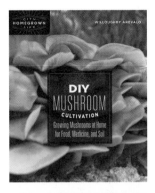

YOU'D LIKE TO be self-sufficient, but the space you have available is tighter than your budget. If this sounds familiar, the **Homegrown City Life Series** was created just for you! Our authors bring country living to the city with big ideas for small spaces. Topics include cheesemaking, fermenting, gardening, composting and, more—everything you need to create your own homegrown city life!

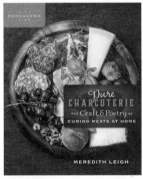

ALSO AVAILABLE

- **The Food Lover's Garden:** *Growing, Cooking and Eating Well* by Jenni Blackmore

- **The Art of Plant-Based Cheesemaking,** revised & updated 2nd edition: *How to Craft Real, Cultured, Non-Dairy Cheese* by Karen McAthy

- **Worms at Work:** *Harnessing the Awesome power of Worms with Vermiculture and Vermicomposting* by Crystal Stevens

- **Pure Charcuterie:** *The Craft and Poetry of Curing Meats at Home* by Meredith Leigh

- **DIY Kombucha:** *Sparkling Homebrews Made Easy* by Andrea Potter

- **DIY Mushroom Cultivation:** *Growing Mushrooms at Home for Food, Medicine, and Soil* by Willoughby Arevalo

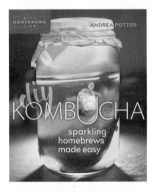

FORTHCOMING

- **Your Indoor Herb Garden** by DJ Herda

- **DIY Sourdough** by John and Jessica Moody

#homegrowncitylife

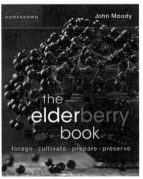

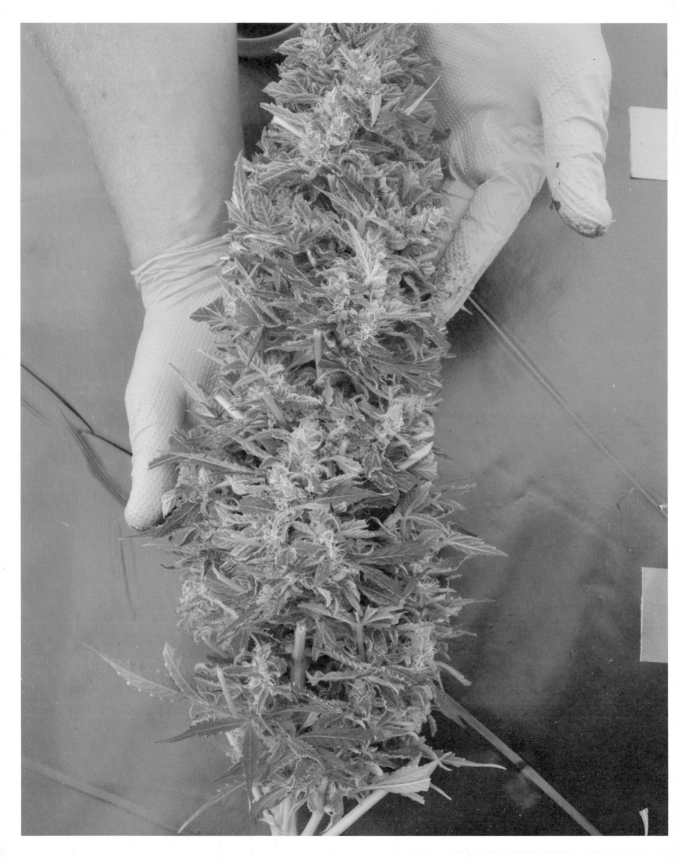

ABOUT THE AUTHOR

J EFF LOWENFELS (Lord of the Roots), is one of the most humorous and entertaining lecturers and writers on the organic
gardening circuit. He is a reformed lawyer who went back
to his childhood roots to become a leader in the organic gardening
movement. He is the author of a series of award-winning and best-
selling books, three of which have become bibles for organic growers
worldwide, including *Teaming with Microbes*, *Teaming with Nutrients*, and *Teaming with Fungi*. Lowenfels has also penned the longest
running garden column in North America and was inducted into the
Garden Writers of America Hall of Fame after serving as President.
He is the founder of Plant A Row for The Hungry, a program which
has resulted in millions of pounds of garden produce being donated
to feed the hungry every year. He lives in Anchorage, Alaska, where
cannabis has been legal since 1975. www.Jefflowenfels.com

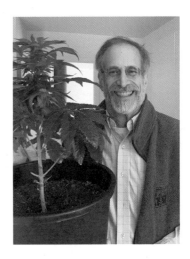

◀ This huge cola from a New Breed
Seed Autoflowering *Cannabis* plant,
Timberline, VAR, is something to strive
for. HAROLD FRAZIER, NEW BREED SEED.

A NOTE ABOUT THE PUBLISHER

New Society Publishers is an activist, solutions-oriented publisher focused on publishing books for a world of change. Our books offer tips, tools, and insights from leading experts in sustainable building, homesteading, climate change, environment, conscientious commerce, renewable energy, and more — positive solutions for troubled times.

We're proud to hold to the highest environmental and social standards of any publisher in North America. This is why some of our books might cost a little more. We think it's worth it!

- We print all our books in North America, never overseas
- All our books are printed on 100% post-consumer recycled paper, processed chlorine free, with low-VOC vegetable-based inks (since 2002)
- Our corporate structure is an innovative employee shareholder agreement, so we're one-third employee-owned (since 2015)
- We're carbon-neutral (since 2006)
- We're certified as a B Corporation (since 2016)

At New Society Publishers, we care deeply about what we publish—but also about how we do business.

 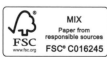

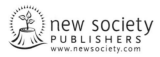

New Society Publishers

ENVIRONMENTAL BENEFITS STATEMENT

For every 5,000 books printed, New Society saves the following resources:[1]

19	Trees
1,752	Pounds of Solid Waste
1,927	Gallons of Water
2,514	Kilowatt Hours of Electricity
3,184	Pounds of Greenhouse Gases
14	Pounds of HAPs, VOCs, and AOX Combined
5	Cubic Yards of Landfill Space

[1]Environmental benefits are calculated based on research done by the Environmental Defense Fund and other members of the Paper Task Force who study the environmental impacts of the paper industry.